The Stranger in the Mirror

A touchingly candid and personal account of lifelong obesity and its emotional, social and physical impact, Ellie Salser takes you on a journey that intimately chronicles her life-changing decision to undergo gastric bypass surgery. Sharing her experiences to the world in the hopes of reaching out to those struggling with weight-related issues, the book is a timeline that begins with the realization and acceptance of her weight problem. Revealing a determination and strength of character that carried Ellie through months of exhaustive research, numerous medical consultations and the difficult decision-making process, the book also details the lengthy preparation, psychological and emotional issues, the surgery, the aftermath and both the positive and negative issues she has dealt with in the 5 years since. It is with great pride that Ellie no longer sees herself as a stranger in the mirror, but a beautiful woman who successfully changed her life.

By Ellie Salser

Copyright © Ellie Salser 2014

The right of Ellie Salser to be identified as the Author of the Work has been asserted by her in accordance with the Copyright, Designs and Patents Act 1988.

All rights reserved; no part of this publication may be reproduced, stored in a retrieval system, or transmitted in any form or by any means, electronic, mechanical, photocopying, recording, or otherwise without the prior written permission of the Author. This book may not be lent, resold, hired out or otherwise disposed of by way of trade in any form of binding or cover other than that in which it is published, without the prior written consent of the Author. No responsibility for loss occasioned to any person or corporate body acting or refraining to act as a result of reading material in this book can be accepted by the Publisher, by the Author, or by the employer(s) of the Author. Certain images copyright.

The names in the book have been changed for privacy reason.

Ellie Salser, The Stranger in the Mirror

This book is dedicated to my father, Brad.

My dad was a loving, sincere man who enjoyed helping others and would do anything for anyone without a second thought. He remained an integral part of my life even though my parents divorced before I was two. Dad picked me up on the weekends and took the time to talk to me on the phone anytime I needed him and continued this even when I grew up. When I visited him either at home or at his mechanic's shop, he stopped whatever he was doing to greet me. If I called when he was with someone, he talked about me with great pride. He showered me with love and made me feel special like every little girl should, and treated his son-in-law and grandchildren the same way. So many people loved and cared about him because he treated everyone with kindness and compassion.

Dad, I'm so proud of you. Thank you for everything you did for me and my family. Now I'd like to do something for you by dedicating this book, to you, my beloved Dad.

Contents

Chapter 1 - The Idea of Weight Loss Surgery - How it All Began

Chapter 2 - Facing Reality

Chapter 3 - The Journey Begins

Chapter 4 - No Turning Back

Chapter 5 - New Beginnings

Chapter 6 - Success

Chapter 7 - Triumphs and Challenges

Chapter 8 - Aftermath

Chapter 1

The Idea of Weight Loss Surgery - How it All Began

It started so innocently, just like so many events that happen when you least expect it. I was at my desk at work talking with my co-workers and friends Amelia and Leah. We worked for a multibillion dollar insurance brokerage firm. It was a great company to work for and the environment was very upscale with plenty of expensive cars in the parking lot and a fairly strict dress code that reflected the ambience. In a sense, Amelia and Leah were more like mentors since both of them were a few years older and more experienced. If I needed advice about anything, work-related or not, they were always there for me, and I have to say they helped me mature in many ways. I enjoyed my job as a graphics designer and looked forward to building a career with the company.

We were certainly a study in contrasts, which made working together so much more interesting.

I was in my mid-twenties, 5'8, about three-hundred pounds, and probably more conservative than many women my age. A natural brunette, I dressed professionally and took care with my hair and makeup. I could be described as a private person, quiet, soft spoken and very sweet.

Amelia was in her mid-thirties and although she seemed on a permanent diet, she had recently lost some weight and it showed. She was 5'7, an attractive and stylish strawberry-blonde who was always beautifully groomed and dressed. You wouldn't have guessed she had three children. Her husband was an accountant and they could enjoy the good life. Even their children's teachers commented that the kids were so well groomed they could be child models.

Leah was a combination of myself and Amelia, was well liked and very creative. She was a brunette about 5'6 and about the half the size of me. She hadn't been married that long but she and her husband had already started a family and purchased a house in a subdivision on the outskirts of town.

Money was the greatest dividing factor between us. I lived with my husband, Allen, and my son, Sam in a starter home on an acre in a rural area of Georgia, so we had to be very frugal. My commute each way to work was forty-five minutes to an hour depending on traffic. Gas money was always put aside when we got paid so we knew we had commuting covered.

Our departmental workload was conducted by hourly timeframes. Producers and their administrative assistants would bring up work that needed to be completed by a specific timeframe. We were at a point where there wasn't anything due for the next few hours so during those downtimes we would visit each other for a chat.

One of the first turning points in my decision to eventually have gastric bypass surgery started off as just another conversation during one of these quiet times. Leah had commented that her sister Joann was always impressed by the fact that Leah always managed to find something to cook even though the fridge was practically empty, whereas Joann could look at the same fridge and find nothing. Leah would pull items from the freezer or straight from the kitchen cabinet and create a great dinner where Joann would give up and think about ordering some food. Leah explained that she liked being creative with whatever she had on hand to make great meals, which impressed Joann.

I told Leah that I also cooked a lot like that since that was how I was taught, and it was something we learned to do when money for food was tight. It wasn't that we went without, but sometimes we had to make do with whatever we had, so I learned to be creative. Leah agreed that it wasn't always the healthiest option as she often fried food or used a lot of butter or cheese.

Amelia's viewpoint was quite different since her husband did most of the cooking, and even when she did cook it was seldom the way Leah or I cooked. Leah then went on to talk about how Joann was dating a guy that had weight loss surgery and how great he was doing. Then she asked if I had ever considered gastric bypass surgery.

There it was … in a single moment, a few words changed my life. Though I managed to say no in what I hoped was a normal voice, I could barely contain the shock and dismay I felt. A couple of minutes ago I was sitting at my desk just like any other day having a normal conversation and suddenly Leah asked me about weight loss surgery. How long had she been wanting to mention it? Did she see me as some obese person desperately in need of help?

I felt my heart sink. Surely only seriously obese people had to take that route, people that were so heavy they were confined to their homes, struggling with health issues or could barely move. That wasn't me. I went to work every day, took care of my appearance and had no major health issues going on. That wasn't who I was … was it? So why did she ask?

After I responded to Leah she stood there sheepishly watching me with an expression that clearly conveyed regret at her words. It upset me even more that she just realized she hurt my feelings. At that point, Amelia suddenly left, though I was so caught up in the awkwardness of the situation I don't remember if someone asked her for help or she just wanted to step away from the situation. Perhaps she wanted to spare me more humiliation because she also thought the question was completely inappropriate.

Too shocked to respond, I tried to focus on checking my email before my emotions got the better of me. I still couldn't believe Leah had asked me such a question, and all I wanted was for her to just go back to her desk and leave me alone. She immediately apologized for upsetting me, but the damage had been done. It went deeper than upsetting me. I honestly never assumed I had that much of a problem with my weight.

As far as I was concerned, I led a normal life and didn't have any medical problems apart from my treatment for postpartum depression. I did have a family history of depression, but it had not affected me until Sam's birth. I wasn't a couch potato stuffing myself with food and at dinner I sat the table with my family. My pants didn't ride up my legs when I walked, and my feet didn't splay because they were too wide for my shoes. I didn't labor for breath when I moved and didn't sweat when I climbed stairs. After all, we couldn't all be one size. Admittedly I didn't like to look at myself in the mirror or go shopping for new clothes, but I wasn't that big ... or was I?

Conflicting emotions churned within me even as I struggled not to think about it. Why did Leah even ask me that question? Did everyone perceive me as someone that needed to lose some serious weight? Did people feel sorry for me because I was heavy? Did I disgust people when they saw me? Had Leah wanted to say something all this time but it just slipped out?

Like an out of control train racing down a track, the thoughts just kept hammering away at me. I knew if I didn't stop my self-destructive thinking I would only make myself depressed and destroy what remained of my self-confidence. I told myself I was beautiful even if I was overweight. There were millions of overweight but attractive and healthy people. Just because someone was overweight didn't mean they needed weight loss surgery ... and so the assurances and excuses continued.

Although I continued with life as usual after the incident with Leah, I did think about whether I was heavy enough for gastric bypass surgery. I didn't constantly dwell on it, nor did I notice any different behavior from others. Everyone treated me the same as always. I was more curious about the possibility of surgery and wondered whether I could actually go through with it. What would my family think? Who qualified for this procedure? What did it entail and was it risky?

After all, I simply needed to lose some extra weight. It wasn't as though my life literally depended on losing weight. Then I considered Leah's comment. Perhaps it hadn't been intended as a cruel remark. Perhaps she simply had my best interests at heart and asked a sincere question as a concerned friend. Regardless, her words stayed in my mind, and so did my thoughts about surgery.

***

Several weeks passed and I treated myself to a new hairstyle. It was above shoulder length and really flattering. I was excited about my new look and was trying out different ways to style it. Looking in a mirror to see the back of my head I noticed that I had back fat. At first I couldn't believe it as I never had back fat before. It actually revolted me out because I thought only really obese people had it.

Was I really that big? Of course not. I just had to lose a little weight and it would disappear. I wasn't in the league of those that needed surgery to lose weight. Suddenly I didn't want to look in the mirror anymore. If I didn't see it, then nobody else would. There was my old friend denial again. Why should I worry? I felt great, had a wonderful husband that loved me and a son I adored. I had family, friends and a good social life. I was the type of person that liked to do things and enjoy life and never spent the day sitting in front of the television. How could I even consider gastric bypass surgery?

If I avoided looking at myself in the mirror from the chest down it was easy to avoid seeing my flaws. What I saw in the mirror was not what I felt like. I felt good. I had a muffin top and I wasn't happy about it but millions of woman had one, including most of the women in my family so it was in my genes. You couldn't control genetics so I simply wore clothes to hide it or didn't draw attention to mid section of my body. My inner thighs also touched but the same went for the other women in my family. It wasn't anything I could control. I never was and never would be a size zero. This was who I was and I had to accept it.

When it came to clothes they served more of a practical purpose for me rather than a fashion statement. I didn't usually like to go shopping because it was always a struggle to find attractive clothes that fit. When you're a plus size your only choices are expensive clothes or a small selection at big box stores, which were seldom a style suited to a younger woman. Finding something I actually liked was hit and miss and if I did manage to find something, buying it depended on whether I could afford it.

When Allen and I got some extra money from our income tax return I decided I needed to get some new clothes since I tended to wear the same clothes all the time. With some extra cash to spend, I knew my best friend, Beth, would help me pick out some cute clothes. It would be morale booster for me and I was excited and really looking forward to shopping and spending the day with my best friend. I usually shopped for clothes alone because I didn't want to have to admit what size I wore, plus when you held up a pair of size twenty-six pants in front of a slim friend, you knew what they were going to think. This time, though, I wasn't going to worry about it. I was just going to have a fun day with my friend and enjoy myself.

We ended up going to a plus size store because I knew we wouldn't find anything at the ordinary clothing stores. For me it was embarrassing to shop there, but it was the only store that offered any kind of variety in my size. Beth was sweet to offer to come with me. Tall and slim, she took great care of herself and always looked amazing. She was around 5'7 and an enviable size 8, but it was the way she dressed and groomed herself that really made her look so glamorous. It wasn't even like she had to spend a lot but because she was a smaller size she had far more options and access to bargains than I did.

Beth and I browsed for a while until I finally found some pants I liked. While trying them on, I noticed that my ankles were red and swollen, almost as though I had edema. The skin didn't feel hot nor did I feel any discomfort, so I realized that my weight and my unsupportive shoes were probably causing my legs to swell. They were brown leather slides with an inch heel that suited either work or casual clothes since I couldn't afford to buy shoes for different occasions.

I was afraid to mention anything to Beth in case she thought something was wrong and suggested I see a doctor. I know that if I noticed her ankles red and swollen like mine I'd be concerned, so I kept it to myself. I just wanted to have a fun day shopping so denial kicked in and convinced me it was just my shoes that had caused the problem, and I simply needed to buy some new ones.

Incidents regarding my weight began to become more frequent, each one serving as a reminder that my denial was my greatest obstacle. Yet another wakeup call occurred when Marie, my sister-in-law, invited my family to watch a football game. She was having a cookout and had invited another couple as well. Everyone was watching the game and having a great time. At half time Marie brought in the barbecue and everyone filled their plates and found a place to sit. Marie and Kevin, her friend's husband, sat at the dining table, which faced the living room where everyone else had already gathered to watch the game.

While trying to adjust myself in the chair, I decided to scoot my chair closer to the table to avoid dropping any barbecue sauce on me. It was a sturdy wooden chair, not some flimsy thing you assembled yourself. When I moved it made a sharp crack like a tree branch snapping off. Marie and Kevin stopped eating and looked at me. The color just drained from my face and I suddenly just wanted to disappear from the embarrassment. Neither of them said or did anything more, but I was so mortified I almost burst into tears.

After that I could barely even look at my food, and I was terrified of moving in case I did break the chair. When the second half of the game started and everyone turned their attention to the television, I told Allen I wanted to leave. I would certainly never want to see Marie's friends again. It didn't help that they were in great shape, which only made me feel worse. Though no one ever mentioned it again, it was yet another memory I had to avoid. Trouble was, there were more and more I had to try and forget about.

What finally chipped away at my stubborn self-denial was when Allen and I went to a race at Talladega Super Speedway with Beth and her husband at the time. They had invited us to go the Nascar event which only occurred twice a year. We also had fantastic seats. The problem was that the seats were quite high, which was great for watching the race, but they were also a challenge to reach and to top it off, I was terrified of heights.

Because the race attracted thousands of fans, we had to park quite a distance away. Walking from the parking lot wasn't bad at all because the grounds were flat, but once we started to climb the stairs, the challenge began. The first few flights weren't bad until I realized I was only about half way up. My breathing became labored, but I didn't want anyone else to notice, especially Allen and my friends. The last thing I wanted was to embarrass him because I couldn't manage a few flights of stairs. I started breathing through my mouth in the hopes of not drawing attention to myself.

When we got about three quarters of the way I noticed a restroom and dashed toward it like I was late for a flight so I could catch my breath. Fortunately no one else was there so I splashed my face with cold water to calm myself down even though I wore makeup. I felt flushed and flustered as I ran water over my wrists as well, and it seemed to take my heart forever to stop pounding.

Of course that made me even more anxious, and if Allen had seen how I labored for breath he would have been embarrassed and concerned for me. I didn't want anyone to know so I stayed in the bathroom until I caught my breath. When I came out Allen was waiting for me and asked if I was all right. Fortunately the others had already gone to their seats, so I told him I just needed to go to the bathroom.

I tried to pace myself as Allen and I climbed to our seats, and once I got settled, there was no way I was coming down or moving for any reason, particularly since I was so afraid of heights. Though the seat locations were fantastic, they had arm rests and for someone overweight, the seats were snug to the point that I soon found myself growing so uncomfortable that I couldn't enjoy the race. I tried to stand most of the time so that I wouldn't have to remain seated, but the poor man behind me couldn't see a thing. Worse, there was a point where I was the only one standing when everyone else was seated.

What was supposed to be an enjoyable evening was becoming a nightmare as it was too uncomfortable for me to sit too long. I worried the entire time about breaking the chair, and I felt guilty for standing and blocking the view of the man behind me. Finally I sat down and he tapped me on the shoulder and thanked me. At that point I was so upset that tears started running down my face. I didn't want to draw attention to myself by crying, especially because Allen was sitting right next to me. I felt so humiliated by yet another situation caused by my weight that instead of enjoying the race, all I could think of was when it ended so I could leave the stands.

Allen noticed my distress and asked if I needed to go the bathroom. I knew if I didn't get out of that seat soon I'd start crying in front of everyone. Once we were in the corridor I opened up to Allen and told him that I was afraid the seat would break and everyone would notice. I had even placed the cooler beneath my seat so that even if it broke it wouldn't be noticeable. Opening up to Allen was like a dam had burst and now all the hurt and frustration came pouring out.

Allen was patient and understanding as always. He assured me that he loved me and would do whatever I wanted. If I wanted to go we'd leave. If not, we'd stay. I told him that I wanted to stay because I didn't want to draw any attention to myself. I didn't think Beth and her husband noticed my distress, but maybe they did and didn't want to mention anything. Preoccupied with thoughts of my weight, I slowly followed Allen back to our seats. I should have been able to enjoy the energy of the crowd and the spectacle of the race but I barely saw or heard anything. When it was finally over I was so relieved to get out of the seat I couldn't wait to leave. At least I had no problems walking down the stairs and getting to the car, but the damage had been done.

All the way back to the car I couldn't stop thinking about my weight. Was it time to consider surgery or did I just have to buckle down and start dieting? Interestingly enough, by the next day I had already started to avoid thinking about my experience at the race and denial started creeping back in. I could always avoid any further problems by simply not attending another race, but this time I couldn't completely brush it off. At night when I tried to sleep, anxieties about my weight and how it was holding me back from enjoying my life plagued me. I wanted to go out and have fun with my friends, but something as simple as sitting comfortably in a chair was just one sign that my weight was a problem, and it was a problem that wasn't going to go away simply by ignoring it.

Why I was so worried about the chair breaking at the race was because of the incident at Marie and one day while attending weight watcher class with Amelia and Leah, I had a chair come apart/break on me during the meeting. We were in a mini college classroom setting and it had stadium style seating. I was about mid way in the seating arrangements. There were only 5 or 6 rows going up and 10 rows going across. In the middle of the rows going up there's a walk way so people can access the seats better and speakers can walk up and hand out flyers, etc. While the weight watchers mentor was passing out handouts, I was sitting on the second seat from the middle and three rows up. She was walking toward me to hand me some papers and I reached over one chair to meet her half way so she didn't have to walk so far. I heard this pop noise and it wasn't load, but the mentor said oh no! Are you ok? And then I realized, the chair had broken on one side. Everyone turned around to look and I was absolutely mortified. I know my face turned red and immediately got a hot feeling go over my body. I wanted to just disappear and wish that it never happened. There were six other people in the room and two of them were Amelia and Leah, thank goodness. I was so embarrassed I didn't want to even look up. I replied yes, I'm ok and just keep my eyes on the floor and just moved to another seat. I didn't look at anyone and I couldn't tell you who they were. I didn't want to know. I stayed for the meeting and acted like it didn't bother me that much. Amelia and Leah both knew that it had hurt my feelings but they didn't say anything. All I could think was why did it have to happen in a weight watchers meeting? It could have been anyone at any meeting and it was me at a weight watchers meeting. I asked Amelia when we got back to our work area what to do about the seat. I didn't want to call maintenance and tell them I broke the seat. I didn't want them asking any questions. Amelia said that she would send them an email just letting them know that it needed to be replaced and they wouldn't ask any questions. I was relieved that she suggested that and it worked out perfectly. I never told anyone about this and it was never spoken of again.

  Maybe it was time to consider having gastric bypass surgery.

  Allen and I finally sat down and discussed the situation. At first I felt awkward, but as I spoke, I felt a sense of relief that at last I was finally admitting that I had a problem. He suggested that we start eating healthier and walking in the afternoon, which would also benefit him because he was also gaining weight. We would tackle the problem together. At this point I had no concerns about health problems because of my age and also because I had checkups every six months as I was on antidepressants.

Though I had started taking antidepressants for postpartum depression, that was no longer the case. Unfortunately I had inherited a tendency toward depression from my mother's side of the family, so when I tried to wean off the medication I became emotional, tearful and irritable very quickly. When I remained on the medication my moods stabilized. At my checkup every six months the doctor took blood work to ensure everything was fine.

I had one son at the time. Since Sam hadn't come to the race with us he was unaware of the problem. No one else knew either as I never spoke about my weight concerns. What did worry me was that I hated dieting. I knew I had to make an effort by trying healthier recipes, but planning weekly meals down to snacks was more effort than I knew I could handle. I still felt that I only needed to lose a little weight and that if I simply buckled down and lost it, I'd reach that goal, maybe not today, but soon enough.

It was interesting how your own thoughts sometimes became your worst enemy. You could talk yourself out of almost anything if you set your mind to it, but fate had a way of throwing obstacles in your path to make you face your demons sooner or later. That decisive moment finally came under the most innocuous of circumstances.

One afternoon I was out with Allen and Sam, it was around four at the time, running errands that included picking up a new light fixture for the house and paying our electricity bill. We also returned a few things to Wal-Mart that we had been putting off. Since we were undecided about what to have for dinner, Sam suggested going to Taco Bell since we all liked their menu. After ordering our food, I went to get a table while Allen and Sam waited at the counter for our order. When I sat down, the chairs and tables bolted onto the floor could not be adjusted and I immediately felt very uncomfortable because I had to really squeeze into the spot to the point where my stomach rubbed against the table. Though I checked the other tables to see if there was different seating, all of the tables and chairs were bolted to the floor and could not be moved.

Suddenly I felt very conspicuous and upset about my situation. While it didn't appear that anyone had noticed, I began to imagine what the others around me might be thinking. I tried to distract myself by looking for my husband and son, who were waiting for our order to be placed on trays and filling drinks at the dispensers. Now my distress and embarrassment grew to the point where I knew there was no way I could bluff my way out of the situation. Allen would immediately notice and if I made a fuss about not wanting to stay, he would ask what was wrong. The last thing I wanted was for him to assume someone had said or done something to upset me, and above all, I didn't want to cause a scene.

When Allen and Sam finally came to the table with the food, I couldn't contain my tears any longer. Allen was clearly distressed and asked me what was wrong and it was all I could do to keep from breaking down in the restaurant. I told him that I was uncomfortable at the table and wanted to leave. He said it would be no problem and went to get the meals boxed up to go, but it was different with Sam, who immediately started asking what was wrong. He thought that I had hurt myself or wasn't feeling well and then asked me if it was because I didn't like the restaurant he picked.

The situation was a pivotal moment in my life. At last I had to face the truth, for how could I possibly explain to my son that his mother was upset because she was to overweight she couldn't fit into the seat at a restaurant table? I made up something to make him feel better, and he responded by hugging me and rubbing my back to comfort me. Of course I never told him anything, but as I walked out of the restaurant, I felt angry and humiliated with myself. Was this the kind of example I wanted to set for my son? Worse, would he pay the price for having an overweight mother, not only socially but with health issues?

On the drive home, I thought about Leah's question regarding gastric bypass surgery. As I watched the passing countryside from the car window, I began to wonder whether it was something I should seriously consider. Suddenly there were so many questions racing through my mind, questions I had asked myself time and time again, but now with more of a sense of urgency. Would I be a suitable candidate? What were the risks and would insurance cover it? What about recovery time? Would it affect my job? I certainly couldn't afford to lose it.

Smelling the food in the bags forced me to question our decision to even go to the restaurant. Clearly, the problem with my weight, and I was finally starting to accept that I did have a problem, stemmed from my background and in the way I viewed food. Though people initially assumed I ate a lot, I actually didn't. I just didn't make smart choices regarding what I ate and didn't eat healthy food. For me, it was about what tasted good. I suppose educating myself about food would have helped me make wiser choices, but I never bothered to consider calories, fat, or actually look at a packaging label. Even if I did, I wouldn't know how to interpret the values since I didn't know the amount of calories I was supposed to have every day.

For me, food was a simple concept. If it tasted good, I ate it. If I didn't like it, I didn't eat it. The sensory appeal of food and feeling satisfied were my main concerns. I wasn't that adventurous with food because we didn't have the money to experiment and if we didn't happen to like something, it would have been a waste of money and meant going without until the next meal. Since that was a mindset I grew up with, I had stuck to it, but now I realized it was a mindset I would have to change, no matter how difficult that process would be.

Chapter 2 - Facing Reality

The holiday season had rolled around and I was enjoying it as I always did. It was my favorite time of the year not only because of the time I was able to spend with my family, but because it was a fun time at work. My little group of friends had gotten together for a photo and I immediately hid behind everyone hoping to conceal as much of my body as possible since most of the other women were rather slim.

Later, when I got my copy of the photo noticed that I was the heaviest in the picture. It was no surprise, but what I didn't realize until I took a good look at the photo was that I was almost the same size as two of the women standing in front of me. The realization of what I saw took a moment to sink in. Looking at Leah standing at the front of the group, I remembered her remark about having weight surgery. It was an awkward moment, and I knew her question was not intended to be hurtful, but after I accepted her apology, we never talked about it again.

Yet now that I looked at the photo with an increasingly critical eye, there was no denying it. Surely I wasn't that big? Every detail stared me in the face. Of course my friend denial kicked in and I decided I wouldn't be displaying the photo.

Again thoughts of the surgery entered my mind, but I told myself I wasn't the right candidate. I was young and had no trouble with mobility. Most likely I wouldn't even qualify for surgery. I had no intention of researching the topic on the computer as well as I didn't want anyone in the office to know about it, and as we couldn't afford a home computer, it was easy for me to put off thinking about it. Of course I could have gone to the library, but again, the chance that someone might see what I was doing was too embarrassing to contemplate.

I managed to put off doing anything about it, but I knew I was simply delaying the inevitable.

***

Allen and I had been married for four years and Sam desperately wanted a brother or sister. It almost became an obsession with him, and since Allen and I definitely planned to have more children, we decided to start trying. At first we were excited and used to stop at the baby section anytime we passed through stores. After several months had passed, our initial excitement transformed into disappointment. Our inability to conceive a child just wasn't happening. I began to worry that the cause might be my weight. I had gotten pregnant with Sam barely a month after Allen and I started trying, and the more had I dwelt on it, the more worried I became.

Doubts plagued me. We had told our family and friends that we were hoping to have another child, but our excitement waned as time passed. In particular, my sister-in-law Marie was so excited that we had decided to have another child. She was already talking about spoiling them and smothering them with love. Her children were a few years older and going through that phase where they didn't like to be hugged or cuddled. Even her body language changed when I told her. We were sitting in the bleachers at Sam's baseball game just chatting. When I told her that Allen and I had discussed having another baby and we were trying, she reached over and embraced me with so excitedly she reminded me of a little girl opening her Christmas presents.

Though her response encouraged me, words alone weren't enough dispel my concern about not being able to conceive. Interestingly, my family has never really brought up my weight. My mother is about an inch taller than me but not as heavy. I once heard my grandmother, who had more of my straight shape; say that my mother was blessed with hips. When my mother and I went shopping, she always suggested that I buy clothes that flattered my curves rather than hide them. But that was easy for someone with a waist and more of an hourglass figure to say. She wasn't in perfect shape, but her figure was different from mine.

    That was probably why I never felt my weight was never an issue. Nobody really made it one, so I didn't think it was that big a deal. The only time I felt overweight is when I saw pictures of myself, my backside in the mirror or when buying clothes. I had no idea how much overweight I was. In my mind it was just a few pounds and if I wanted to lose it then I could.

    I remember how my initial response to Marie's delight faded into self-doubt and worry. Had I told everyone about our plans to have another baby too soon? Now I started to really worry. Was it God's plan for us to have only one child? I was starting to get depressed about my inability to get pregnant to the point where I donated the baby items I have saved. I started with the small items first, then as time went on I donated or sold the larger items. Three years passed and I still couldn't conceive.

    Finally, I faced reality and talked to my doctor about my concerns. During past checkups he had briefly discussed my weight, but it was the in general terms the way all doctors tended to unless you were in perfect shape. He told me there could be several reasons why I wasn't able to conceive, and when I asked if it could be my weight, he agreed that could be one of the reasons.

    I recalled several conversations with Amelia and Leah in which they had also mentioned that their doctors advised them to lose weight even though they weren't that overweight. Well, no one needed to tell me what I already knew. Discussing weight and smoking with patients was almost like a mantra, but at least I didn't smoke, so that was at least one less concern.

    As for my depression, that was more from family history than weight gain. If I became upset after skipping my medicine for a few days, it wasn't because of my weight but usually something insignificant like a spill or burnt toast. Of course no one should really stress over insignificant issues, and if I stayed on my medication the small upsets weren't a problem anymore ... but it seemed my weight was one problem that wasn't going to go away simply because I ignored it.

I desperately wanted to have a baby. I didn't want to have surgery and then get pregnant. It made no sense to have weight loss surgery then gain it back after having a baby. Once again I thought about researching the surgery. If my weight was preventing me from having a baby, it was up to me and only me to take steps to change the situation. No one else was going to do it for me, and I understood that I had avoided the truth as long as I could.

So I finally researched what I could about gastric bypass surgery. It was an interesting experience to finally face those demons of denial. I essentially had two choices, either gastric bypass surgery or lap band. The lap band procedure required a port in the stomach for injections, which made me extremely uncomfortable. I certainly didn't like the thought of a port in my stomach and wondered if it would be uncomfortable if I moved the wrong way. Would it be prone to infection or need regular maintenance? And the thought of shots really didn't sit well with me. I decided to pass on this option.

That left gastric bypass surgery. But that was major surgery, and that worried me even more than shots. What if something happened? I had a son and would leave my wonderful husband and family behind. Would it be worth risking my life for weight loss surgery? I realized I was scaring myself before I even knew the facts and whether I would even be a suitable candidate.

I did my best to put aside my fears and continued researching. When I discovered I fell into the morbidly obese category I was frankly quite stunned. How was that possible? The word alone sounded like something horrible. Surely I didn't fall in this category? I felt the face of denial rearing its ugly head and prompting me to check other sites since I couldn't possibly morbidly obese.

Another site I found indicated that a BMI of 40 BMI was considered morbidly obese. This meant I had to figure out if I fell into this category, so when I found a BMI calculator for females and reviewed my results, I was beyond devastated. Not only was I morbidly obese, but my BMI index was 52.46, class 3 obese. I remember simply staring at the screen like a deer caught in headlights. Could it possibly get any worse? I was over 40 BMI by 12.46%.

Maybe it would time to take a really good look at myself in the mirror as my self-esteem just hit rock bottom. I kept reading the same sentence over again about class 3 obesity, which put me at an extremely high risk of weight-related disease and premature death. It was important that I see a doctor to get help for my condition … but what condition? I was just overweight. How was that a critical condition? What would a doctor do or tell me that I didn't already know or could do myself? I mean, I couldn't be morbidly obese even though my BMI was 52.46. Who came up with that number anyway? It was easy to throw out figures. Truth was, I didn't need a number to make me feel guilty about being overweight. I was doing a fine job on my own.

I needed time to process what I had just discovered and understand the implications. It could have been denial trying to cast doubt about the information, but the internet was simply a mediator, an impartial source that only provided information. It didn't judge, it didn't assess, it was just an impartial source of facts, facts that I had actively sought out. This was a reality I had to face whether I wanted to believe it or not. The facts were there in black and white. Could this be why I couldn't get pregnant? It was the question I was afraid to ask yet yearned to answer.

***

It was now over three years since Allen and I had been trying to conceive a child and I finally skipped a period. Could I finally be pregnant after all this time? With a sense of anticipation I made an appointment to see my ob/gyn. I didn't bother to buy a pregnancy test this time because when I was pregnant with Sam it showed negative, so I didn't feel I could trust the results. Once I saw Dr. Jones' face I knew immediately the news wasn't good, which he confirmed when he told me I wasn't pregnant.

I did my best to swallow my disappointment. Dr. Jones was a respected and experienced doctor who treated my mother, aunts, cousins and my friends as well. He was renowned for delivering babies throughout central Georgia. I suppose if you imagined a Norman Rockwell type of a doctor, Dr. Jones would be the perfect subject. He was warm, had a great sense of humor and his caring demeanor instilled confidence. You knew that he would help you to the best of his abilities, or he would refer you to someone that could.

I was beyond disappointed since I had never missed a period before. Dr Jones explained that there could be a number of reasons why I had skipped a period and told me he could give me a shot to help regulate my cycle or I could just wait until next month to start. I didn't want a shot, I wanted answers and asked him if my weight could be the issue. He told me it was a strong possibility.

Well, there it was. I had danced around the issue long enough so I finally asked if I had weight loss surgery, could I have a baby afterward? Dr. Jones responded with so much enthusiasm that I felt like he had been simply waiting for the moment to discuss it. He thought it was a great idea and that I could have a baby later when I was ready. I wondered why he was so excited that I was considering this surgery but then he went on to explain that he knew several people that had the surgery and it was a wonderful tool to help people lose weight.

At first I was a little taken aback. If he thought it was such a great idea why hadn't he mentioned it before? Then it occurred to me that weight was a sensitive subject to people. Even now I had my doubts, so if he'd asked me about it before I probably would have been very defensive. Undoubtedly that was one reason why he was so popular because he never nagged about weight. And dealing with only women all these years must have also taught him how to be diplomatic and not tick off his patients.

My general doctor, Dr. Powell, had mentioned it briefly to me, but when he asked if I'd ever considered weight loss surgery, I told him I didn't want to do anything that drastic. That was the end of that conversation and I never gave the suggestion another thought until Leah mentioned it.

When I went to see Dr. Powell for my routine checkup, I mentioned that I was considering weight loss surgery. He absolutely loved the idea and told me it would be a great decision to help me lose weight. Clearly, both my doctors agreed that weight loss surgery would be ideal for me. It seemed that simply losing weight wasn't the option I had hoped, but surgery seemed to be. Still, I wasn't certain. I needed more information, more time to make an informed decision.

Dr. Powell referred me to a group of weight loss doctors in the building and told me they were a great team. I have to admit his eagerness was disconcerting. After discovering that I was considered morbidly obese, I hadn't bothered to do much further research and I was frankly curious why he liked the idea so much. My appointment with Dr. Powell was an opportunity to get a second opinion about the weight loss surgery. He suggested that I make an appointment to talk to them.

After that, I realized I had to be better informed before I could even think about making a decision, so I continued my research. The team of doctors that Dr. Powell and Dr. Jones recommended had glowing reviews and the website provided all the information I needed about the surgeons, the review process, the procedure and a section for general questions that was very helpful. I did see that hair loss was a possible side effect but I could still have a baby within one to two years of surgery.

I particularly liked that the website didn't say anything negative about being overweight. It provided facts and different options available to improve your health, and I could even attend a free seminar conducted by the bariatric staff and surgeons who gave a presentation about the process and the different options. Here was my opportunity to finally address my concerns and question.

At this point Allen was the only other person I had talked to about my weight issues. When I first mentioned that that was thinking about surgery, he was initially concerned for my safety. He told me he loved me the way I was, but if I wanted to go ahead with the surgery he would support my decision. He also expressed the same concerns as mine about the surgery, so I told him I was thinking about attending the seminar. He agreed it would be a good idea and wanted me to be as informed as possible about the procedure before making a decision. The next seminar was in two weeks so I signed up and decided to be prepared by doing as much research as possible.

I returned to the website to read further about recovery time, which was different depending upon the procedure you chose. The more

I read about the lap band the more anxious I became as I didn't want to stomach port, but the benefit was a much quicker recover than gastric bypass surgery. Lap band recover ranged from one to three weeks, while gastric bypass recovery was three to six weeks. That was a long time for me to be off work.

There were pros and cons for both procedures. Bypass surgery weight loss would bring you to your weight loss goals to within about a year, but lap band would take longer. I was leaning more toward bypass surgery, but I was concerned about the hair loss that was common during the third through eleventh month post-surgery because of rapid weight loss. The thought of losing more hair bothered me as I was losing enough already, I certainly didn't want bald patches all over my scalp. Other risks included leakage around the staple line where the new pouch was formed, or tears or rips in the area. Blood clots were a risk that could occur with any surgery, not just weight loss surgery.

I tried to keep reading but the list of complications continued. Blood clots could be prevented by getting up and moving around within four hours after surgery, but that sounded terribly painful. Another risk was wound infections, a problem that occur if wounds weren't kept clean. At least I knew that I could handle that one. Following the prescribed diet and not smoking two weeks before surgery also reduced the risks. I didn't smoke so that wouldn't be a problem, and the diet also seemed like something I could follow as it was high in protein and low in fat, sugar, fiber and carbohydrates. That would be easy enough to follow for two weeks since I loved cheese, eggs and meat. Vitamins and supplement were important, and included multivitamins, B-12 and calcium, and I was already taking multivitamins now, so that was another item I could check of the list of concerns.

When I saw the downsides of the bypass surgery it was hard for me to contain my anxiety. Nausea and vomiting was the most common complications occurring in the first few months after gastric bypass surgery. I wondered how bad that would be and how long those symptoms would last. It could happen after eating too fast, drinking liquids while eating, not chewing enough, or eating more than the pouch can comfortably hold. It was important to learn to eat very slowly and thoroughly chew food. Nausea and vomiting could also be triggered after trying new foods. If that occurred it would be necessary to wait a few days before trying a new food again.

    Clearly, I was going to have to learn how to eat and drink all over again. I didn't eat fast, but I did drink while I ate. Then there was dehydration. Your pouch could only hold three to four ounces, so you need to drink more often because there was less room to hold fluids. That I could probably handle as well. I was more concerned by Dumping Syndrome, which happened when food passed through the stomach too fast into the small intestines. Symptoms included a combination of nausea, uncomfortable fullness, cramping, diarrhea, weakness, sweating, and fast heart rate. Dumping was provoked by eating very sweet or sugary foods. Of course the greatest issue was overeating.

    I had to take a break from all the thoughts and concerns buzzing through my head. Could I really do all this? Well, I was morbidly obese and I didn't get this way by not eating. So I was going to have to suck it up and take the bad news. Almost everyone requiring gastric bypass surgery have had problems with overeating. The causes for this were complex but involved genetics, emotions, upbringing, and even the functions of the brain. None of this changed after bypass surgery, except that the stomach was much smaller. Eating more than the new stomach can hold cold cause vomiting, expansion of the pouch, weight gain, or even rupture of the stomach. Education, counseling, group support, and certain medications could help prevent overeating and were just as important as diet to the success of the operation.

    Everything was worded neutrally and diplomatically. Never once did I feel like I was a fat slob with no self control. I still didn't believe that I ate that much, but rather, what I ate. Was my old friend denial stopping by to say hello? Not this time. I continued reading, and now more complications came to light, including stomach pain, ulcers, and gastritis (an inflammation of the stomach lining), which would require medical attention after having bypass surgery. Now that made me nervous.

    Then I realized up until now I'd been focusing on myself, me, my fears, my concerns. What about my family?

    Though Allen and I discussed weight loss surgery, he never considered himself a candidate. I was more overweight then him and like me, he didn't think the issue was that bad. He was carrying some extra weight but at 6'2, he was a big, broad-shouldered man. Many people assumed because of his size that he had played football in high school and possibly played in college. Allen was from a small town in Missouri and they didn't have football in the town that he grew up in. Basketball and Baseball is the main sports there, so that's what sports he was involved in.

Sam was built like his dad. He was quite tall for his age maybe twenty pounds overweight. He slimmed down and then got chunky right before another growth spurt. His doctor never mentioned any health concerns as Sam had always been off the charts with height and weight for his age group. None of us had any health problems, but I did want Sam to be better informed about eating healthier. Just like any parents that wanted more for their children than they had, I wanted my son be knowledgeable about calories, carbs, protein, fiber, and nutrition in general. Yes, everyone knew that burgers and fries weren't healthy choices, but I wanted him to be able to look at a label and make educated decisions.

If I wanted that for my son, then only I could set that example for him to follow.

Chapter 3 - The Journey Begins

  I went ahead and officially signed up for the seminar. For several minutes I stared at the screen after I filled out the information as my mind swirled with questions, doubts and uncertainties. Once I submitted the form, I was committing myself to something long-term and life changing. I was nervous and excited, but also a little scared. Would I be able to follow through? Did I have what it took to face this challenge? I had read the success stories and testimonials, but I had also read stories about failure. Would my story eventually be read by others facing the same issues with their weight? Finally, I submitted the form.

  Because I enrolled for the seminar online, no one else besides Allen knew about my decision to attend. At times it was difficult to keep everything inside, but I honestly felt too embarrassed to tell anyone. This way I didn't have to listen to everyone's comments and opinions, and when it came to weight, everyone had an opinion. I'd always been a private person, but in this case I could only imagine the negative responses and I didn't want to open the door to an avalanche of uneducated advice. It was enough that I faced a life-changing decision, but I needed the time and space to make an informed decision based on the facts rather than hysteria.

Somehow time seemed to fly once I received confirmation about the seminar. Allen asked if I wanted him to come with me but I told him I preferred to go alone. It was important that I did this by myself as I wanted to be able to walk away if I got uncomfortable with the situation and not have to deal with the fallout from others knowing about it. I told him that I would be fine going alone. It was just a meeting and there wasn't really anything he could do to help me, but I would let him know if I changed my mind. He was fine with it, but said it would be no problem if I changed my mind and wanted him to attend.

Since the seminar was scheduled at a local hospital during the middle of the day, it worked perfectly for me. I could take an extended lunch and return to work afterward. I left work early enough to arrive at the seminar without rushing as I didn't want to walk into a room full of people and struggle to find a seat. The hospital was bustling and barely anyone noticed me as I made my way to the conference room hosting the seminar. It was my plan to blend in with crowd in case anyone I knew happened to be there. I would stay long enough to see how the meeting went, but I wanted to sit by the aisle in case I felt uncomfortable and wanted to make a quick getaway.

I thought I'd be more nervous, but then it kicked up a notch when I entered the conference room filled with about fifty overweight people. It was pleasant, high-ceilinged room with a projection screen set up at the front. Behind a podium and microphone, a nurse's assistant sat at a table sorting papers. At first it was disconcerting to be surrounded by so many obese people. Even though I was the youngest, all ages, as well as nationalities, were represented. Some people had difficulty walking and used canes and walkers as I expected. Some were well dressed and others some were not. Some had insurance while others had none, so although the group was small, it was diverse.

Seeing others in worse condition than me helped put my own concerns into perspective. While there was some conversation, I sensed that everyone else was a little anxious about their options.

I found an end of row seat on the right side of the room about a third of the way back. There were a few women in front of me and a couple behind me. Now the room was really starting to fill up. A man sat beside me and tried starting a conversation with me but I really didn't want to talk, and certainly not about why I was there. Frankly, I didn't want to share my story with a stranger. I knew why I was there and I didn't really want to discuss how my inability to control my eating habits brought me to a room filled with others equally unable to control their weight. I discreetly let him know that I didn't want to talk and hoped the meeting would start soon.

    Finally the bariatric coordinator stepped up to the podium and introduced herself as Margaret as she began speaking. Instantly the room fell into an expectant hush. In a friendly, conversational tone, she did a great job answering questions before starting the presentation. Everyone seemed to have the same concerns that I did, and I found my comfort level gradually increasing as others voiced my thoughts. I was far from alone in my situation, and I realized I would never be.

    After Margaret spoke, Dr. Johnson, one of the surgeons from the website, stepped up to the podium and introduced himself. He told us he was with Bariatric Surgeons at the hospital and announced his partner's names in the same practice. He then outlined the two different options available and went into more detail about them. People from the audience were very excited to ask him questions, and he often stopped throughout the presentation to make sure everyone had a chance to address their concerns before proceeding. I have to admit it was very interesting and informative.

    Using a slide show presentation, Dr. Johnson showed pictures of how the surgery would be performed and what he would be doing in fairly graphic detail. He said that it would be up to the individual to decide which procedure would be the best for them. No matter how many questions anyone asked, Dr. Johnson answered each one. The more he spoke, the more confident I felt about him, his team and the procedure. I was still leaning toward gastric bypass surgery because weight loss was quicker and I could avoid the port. Now and again I looked at the others to gauge their reactions. Clearly some were convinced while others looked uncertain. It would have taken some element of courage to come here and face the reality of making a positive change in their lives, but at least now we knew we would have all the support we needed.

Once Dr. Johnson finished his presentation, Margaret returned and fielded more questions. Many questions regarded insurance and payment methods. Some insurance companies required candidates to complete a documented six-month diet plan, while some companies required nothing at all. The coordinator emphasized that each visit had to be paid at each appointment and then the insurance company would reimburse the amount. That didn't make a lot of sense to me since I paid insurance to avoid paying anything up front. I was going to have to ask more about this when the time came.

Margaret told us there was a sign up sheet in the back of the room to make appointments with the surgeons for consultations, and that the cost would be $200 for the first visit. Suddenly it was almost like a stampede as people started getting up and rushing toward the sign up sheet. I had never seen overweight people move so fast before. By the time I got to the sign in sheet it was almost a three-month wait to see the surgeon, so I made an appointment. Once the appointment was made I received a checklist of items I needed to bring. I had to collect all information, including the last five years of health records, to prove that I had been overweight for several years. I also had to start a documented, six-month diet plan. Reading over the checklist as I returned to my car, I realized I had my work cut out for me.

At work, I called my insurance company to see if they covered the surgery and what I needed to do to get started. In addition to proving that I had been over 40 BMI for the last five years, I had to undergo a mental evaluation, EKG and several other tests before I could be approved. I also had to get a recommendation from another doctor, so I asked my Dr. Powell for that. Dr. Powell was happy to hear that I had contacted Bariatric Surgeons and was happy to give me a written recommendation. He mentioned that I had no idea how much this was going to help me in the long run. I would avoid joint problems later in life as I wouldn't be carrying around so much weight, not to mention help my heart and other organs.

His enthusiasm reassured me that I was making the best decision for my health and I was starting to feel more and more confident about the surgery. That my doctors were both so excited really made a significant impact on me. Their support was critical during this stage and I knew at that point I was heading in the right direction.

The first step on the list was starting my documented diet, so I attended weekly meetings to weigh in. It was the Weight Watchers plan that required a weekly meeting and weigh-in. The detail of each weigh-in was documented on a small card. Since I had tried this program before I knew what the meetings entailed so I just weighed in and left. All I needed was a dated signature with the date and my weight.

This way everything was documented and I didn't have to rely on anyone else to keep up with it. I had to attend meetings for three consecutive months to satisfy the insurance company's requirements. For me the process was tedious and I didn't like staying for the meetings as the group leaders always invited me to stay and I never wanted to. To get around this I started going to other locations and when they realized that I wasn't staying for the meetings, I returned to the original location.

I know it was somewhat sneaky, but by going to different locations I was able to simply weigh in and get documented, which was the most important thing to me. I started to feel guilty about not staying for the meetings but I just wasn't interested. Though the program was effective, I always felt like I was starving. After a few weeks I'd give in and eat everything I could get my hands on, so this time around I was going along with the program only for the documentation. I knew the process and how to work the system. Paying twelve dollars a week was much cheaper than paying full price for the surgery, and it was a requirement I needed to meet before I could meet the surgeon. When I first started the program my maximum weight was three hundred and thirty-five pounds. Yes, I was aware how high that number was, especially for a young woman that didn't consider herself overweight.

One of the audience members at the seminar asked whether following the Weight Watchers program to lose weight and then gaining it back would still be covered by insurance. The coordinator responded by saying that everyone was encouraged to do their best to be healthy, but if anyone lost weight following the Weight Watchers program, and the insurance company knew you were successful then they would not pay for the surgery. If someone was unsuccessful then they would cover the surgery because if the diet plan failed to help, surgery would be a better option.

It was evident the coordinator didn't want to mention this but I believe that she wanted to be honest because she had seen patients lose weight and then not be approved for surgery. So if someone lost five pounds the first week, which most people did because water weight was the first to shed, you couldn't really lose too much weight. You would have to stay at the same weight or maybe fluctuate a pound or two. It sounded like a contradiction, but not losing weight seemed to guarantee approval for surgery.

Of course if anyone happened to have $4,000 - $5,000 to pay for the surgery then there was no requirement to follow the diet plan anyway. It was a tedious process but I stuck with it. Getting the paperwork from my doctors to prove I had been overweight for five years was an easier task. I was able to go to Dr. Jones and Dr. Powell to get copies of my records from all my annual visits so that was another item checked off my list.

When I finally I attended my first meeting with the surgeon I remember how I thought the three-month diet prerequisite seemed like an eternity, yet now as I drove to my appointment, I felt the same swirl of emotions, doubts and concerns. On my way to his office, which was located at the hospital, a stream of questions played through my mind. What exactly did the procedure entail? Where would the incisions be made, how many and how large? How much of my stomach would remain? The more I thought about the surgery, the more details I wanted to know.

Then I started worrying about the waiting room. Would everybody be there for weight loss surgery or just surgery in general? I wondered if people would notice me and ask questions, which I wasn't ready to answer. Worse, I hoped I wouldn't run into someone I knew at the hospital, because at that point they were bound to ask questions I definitely didn't want to answer. Then again, I could have been there for a checkup. Why was I even worrying so much about what others thought?

Then my thoughts turned to the chairs in the waiting room. I was really on a roll today. Hopefully they weren't too close together because I didn't want to touch anyone else, and when you had a heavy person sitting beside another, that was inevitable. I also thought about how much I was I going to have to pay upfront for other tests because I was worrying about paying too much out of pocket.

Okay... it was time to turn off the voice screaming inside my head. I parked and made my way to the fifth floor. Fortunately, Dr. Reed was running on time so I literally walked in the door, filled out the paperwork and was called in almost immediately, which was a pleasant surprise considering the waits I was used to. Though the office was small, it was clean, professional, and nicely decorated. There were fifteen chairs, including some bench style, others with and without arms, so the seating turned out to be no problem at all.

I quickly realized that this team of doctors performed not only weight loss surgery, but dealt with gall bladder and colon surgery, as well thyroid and lymph node biopsies and a variety of other procedures. There was no way to know why I was there, and I no longer felt self-conscious because the other patients were clearly there for other reasons, not just for weight loss surgery.

When I was called into Dr. Reed's office, the nurse took my weight and blood pressure and told me the doctor would be in shortly. It was a typical examination room with a counter filled with brochures and informational packets. After a few minutes Dr. Reed came in and introduced himself. I was immediately comfortable with him. Pleasant, easygoing and with an easy smile, it was almost as though we had met for coffee as he talked to me like a person rather than a patient. He asked me if I decided which surgery I wanted, so I told him I was leaning toward gastric bypass instead of the Lap Band.

He then proceeded to a white board on the back of the door and used markers to draw diagrams as he spoke about the procedure. I was to stop him any time to ask questions. There were five incisions less than a half an inch long, and that the stomach was cut and sewn back to reduce the size. What was cut off was not removed because it retained blood flow and was still viable, so in case of complications, the stomach could be restored to its original size.

I had always assumed what was cut off from the stomach was removed and asked what would happen if I need to revert to the original size for any reason. Dr. Reed assured me that the odds were very low of that happening. Then I asked how often patients returned after eating too much and bursting their stomachs. He said it was a rare occurrence, but gave me an example of a man who went straight to a drive thru right after leaving the hospital and ate several cheese burgers. Of course his stomach ruptured and he was rushed back into surgery to repair it. I shook my head at that one. How could someone go through the ordeal of weight loss surgery and then do something so stupid? Dr. Reed had no answer to that, but he stressed that it was a rare occurrence for someone to overeat before the stomach had time to heal properly. He talked to me like I was his friend in a language that I could I understand rather than using medical terms to make himself feel superior. His goal was to explore my concerns were and to thoroughly answer my questions no matter how embarrassing or awkward they might be. He was there to provide me information just as I was providing him with information.

    I found him very likable. He was smiling, upbeat and proudly showed off his latest tablet. I even asked him about it since I'd never seen one like it before and he took the time to demonstrate it for me. He was certainly well-dressed beneath his doctor's coat and even the casual way he sat on his swivel stool conveyed a relaxed, easygoing demeanor. I think we were both assessing each other to determine if I would be a good patient and he would be a good doctor.

    Next came questions about any health issues. I explained that I only took antidepressants, which Dr. Reed assured me wouldn't be a problem. I also mentioned that a psychiatric exam was on my checklist, and he explained that part was important because it determined if I could handle the emotional consequences of weight loss surgery. A psychologist would have to approve me but I told him that it wouldn't be an issue. True, I had wrestled with doubts and anxieties for some time, but the fact that I was talking with him was a milestone for me. Above all, I was truly impressed by his credentials, of which bariatric surgery was only one of his specializations. Between his expertise and years of experience, I felt that he would be an excellent choice as my surgeon.

    It turned out that I was an excellent candidate for the surgery. Dr. Reed felt confident that I would do well since I didn't suffer from high risk conditions such as sleep apnea or high blood pressure. In fact, my risk of complications was below the normal range, which made me feel even more confident since that meant I had less than a one percent chance of suffering complications or death during surgery. Well, there it was, the last question I wanted to ask but didn't really want to hear about, but I finally asked him to explain exactly what that meant. First, he reassured me that this question was universal regarding surgery as with every surgery there was a risk of death from complications. Some patients were also difficult to anesthetize, but since I didn't fall into a high-risk category, he was able to ease my concerns.

By the end of the appointment I felt almost liberated. Not only had I gone farther with my weight loss goals than ever before, but I had reached a point where I could resolve my weight issue once and for all. I was proud that I had overcome my self-imposed limitations and was finally able to accept that I had weight problem and be willing to overcome this challenge. Certainly, my doctors would be delighted to know I had opted to have the surgery. All I had to be diligent about was changing my eating habits and avoid stretching my pouch after surgery.

At the conclusion of the appointment Dr. Reed asked if I had any other questions and I told him he had been more than helpful. He said he would be available to address any other concerns and referred me to the bariatric nurse to schedule my EKG and take care of any other information necessary to start my file. Interestingly enough, it was Margaret, the nurse had been the speaker at the seminar that had introduced Dr. Johnson. Now I felt even more comfortable. She asked me which surgery I had decided to choose and I told her gastric bypass. Next she asked if I had talked to my insurance company, which I had, and gave her their list of requirements. I also told her that I was finishing my weekly diet program, and I was very encouraged when she said I was doing extremely well and to continue what I was doing. With the progress I'd made, I'd be approved for the surgery in no time.

Margaret then gave me a binder entitled, 'Toolkit for Gastric Bypass Surgery.' It was a comprehensive guide outlining everything from the contact information for Bariatric Surgeons to detailed lists including a patient accountability guide of pre-operative requirements, insurance requirements, out of pocket expenses, and another checklist. Margaret had placed color-coded tabs on pages to help me stay organized. The first tab highlighted insurance information, then pre-op testing appointments, physical therapy exercises, bariatric support group, pre-op and post-op diet and instruction, journal, resources and information supporting what Dr. Reed had already discussed with me.

She also provided a list of thrift stores in different counties where clothes too big after surgery could be donated. In addition, this section provided a list of gyms, workout centers and Curves locations in the area. A miscellaneous tab listed locations selling high protein supplements. The last tab was the best, and got me really excited because there was a place for you to post photos of yourself during your journey. It not only provided me with a comprehensive source of information I needed and some I hadn't even thought of yet, but it provided me inspiration and the motivation to meet my goals.

The binder became part of me as I carried it with me every day. I did change the cover to 'Believe, Hope, Faith, and Happiness' so no one would know what it was ... at least for the time being. I left the office full of pride and confidence in myself for meeting a difficult challenge and not giving up. Margaret told me she would be happy to assist me in any way. I had successfully completed my first visit to Bariatric Surgeons, and it was more than worth the $200 payment. I had invested in my health and my life ... and who could put a price on that?

When I got home Allen very curious to know what happened and what decision I had made. We got comfortable in the living room, he on the recliner and me on the couch beside him so we could face each other. I relayed what Dr. Reed and I had discussed and Allen agreed that it was the best choice for me. I told him about Margaret had everything organized and ready for their patients, which also impressed me since that showed they were prepared and well organized. I felt that everything was falling into place and that the process was going far more smoothly than I ever imagined.

I reassured Allen by mentioned Dr. Reed didn't feel I had any red flags regarding to surgery and was confident I would be the ideal patient and that my recovery would go well. I knew I could deal with the surgery and recovery, and the only issue that still concerned me was whether I would be able to lose the weight. Admittedly, I wanted to share my success story, and I wanted to lose the weight once and for all and keep it off. Allen never said a word, but listened and watched me carefully. I knew I was speaking from my heart, and all the doubts and excuses I'd lived with for so many years were finally clearing like the aftermath of a storm.

Finally, Allen agreed that it sounded like it would be a great surgery for me and that he felt I was on the right track. He asked if I had any concerns, but I told not only had they all been addressed, but that I was actually starting to get excited about the surgery! However, I still had to meet the approval qualifications for the insurance company, because to pay for the procedure was otherwise impossible as it was well beyond our budget. The $200 for my first appointment with Dr. Reed was pushing our budget as it was, but Allen had always been very supportive of me and never complained about the cost.

I think the greatest quality Allen possessed was his loving, affectionate nature. He was not afraid to express it or show it, whether it was, "Good morning, beautiful," kissing or holding my hand in the car, or a hundred other little details that made our relationship so special. We were happy together and could always talk honestly and openly about any subject. I could always rely on him to be truthful and give me an honest opinion even though it wasn't what I always wanted to hear, but that's what strengthened our relationship. He is a wonderful man, a loving husband and father. I couldn't ask for someone better, and I realized how truly fortunate I was to have Allen in my life.

Chapter 4 - No Turning Back

The next step involved undergoing a psychiatric exam to ensure I was mentally capable of accepting all the emotional factors that came with the surgery and the change of lifestyle it entailed. I was nervous about the evaluation because I thought everyone had a little instability, but mainly because I took two antidepressants daily and I was concerned that my condition might be deemed a negative when I went to meet Dr. Stewart. I was actually more concerned about how much this visit was going to cost as I took an extended lunch. Fortunately, all the doctors were locally fairly close to where I worked in downtown Atlanta.

When I turned into the plaza where the office was located, I wasn't sure that I was in the right place even though I had used MapQuest to obtain directions. Located near a now vacant plaza where I had taken computer classes some years ago, it was backed by a residential area. I finally found the entrance after walking around and spotting the suite number on a discreet sign. Of course I had decided to wear heels on a day when I wasn't just parking and riding up in an elevator.

The moment I stepped into the waiting room I felt that familiar anxiety grip me even though the room was larger and less crowded than Dr. Reed's waiting room. I started feeling self conscious but then I forced myself to snap out of it. No one here knew me and I could have been there for any reason. It was time to change my mental attitude as much as my eating attitude if the surgery was going to be a success for me. Putting my concerns about everyone else behind me, I completed the paperwork and paid $75 up front since insurance hadn't yet started covering these visits.

    Despite my efforts to remain calm, that little voice started nagging from the back of my mind. I started wondering if I was making the right decision. In truth I was very uncomfortable talking to strangers about my weight and began fidgeting in my chair. My throat had gotten so dry I had to ask for some water, and I realized I had to get a grip on my anxiety.

    Shortly after returning the paperwork, I was called into Dr. Stewart's office. The room was comfortably furnished with a couch and had the typical ambience you expected in a psychiatrist's office. I sat on the couch and she sat across from me in a chair. Dr. Stewart was a very sweet, attractive and well-dressed brunette who reminded me of Laura Bush. Her demeanor instantly made me feel at ease. She started the session by asking me numerous questions, including why I wanted to have the surgery and whether I had told my family. I explained why I wanted to have the surgery, which I thought would be self explanatory, but I answered as best I could even though I chafed at having to go into such detail.

    Frankly, I didn't want to have to deal with such personal questions, but I understood that I wanted to be approved for the surgery I had no choice but to respond as honestly as possible. The more cooperative I was, the sooner I could put this visit behind me, so I explained that I wanted to play with my child without getting tired or out of breath. I wanted to be able to get out of the floor without having to grab or pull something. Also, I wanted to wear clothes that I didn't have to adjust all day or made me feel like people were disgusted by my appearance. Above all, I wanted to have another child, and by losing weight, that could become a reality. That response seemed to resonate most with Dr. Stewart.

    Her next focus was on why I hadn't told more of my family. Now I had reason to pause. Why hadn't I told my parents? I suppose I wanted to wait until I knew I was definitely going ahead with the surgery. Once I opened that door, everyone would have an opinion and the endless debates and discussions would start. I saw no point since I hadn't made a final decision myself, plus I had to know the insurance would approve the surgery. My father would be fine with my decision apart from asking the usual questions about the safety and success of the procedure, but my mother was another story. She would be constantly worrying about my decision to have elective major surgery as opposed to surgery I needed to save my life.

I loved both my parents very much but they have different personalities and I wasn't ready to talk to them about this yet. Dr. Stewart picked up on my hesitation and suggested I tell them, and I told her that I would consider discussing it with them. I knew they cared about me and would want the best for me, and it was really was just a matter of timing for me. Her other questions were mostly the typical you'd expect and the appointment was only an hour, which I didn't consider long enough considering the $75 I had to pay since the insurance didn't cover the evaluation. Once again I couldn't help wonder how much Dr. Stewart made in the course of just one day. I would have been happy to have a well-paid job like hers.

Another requirement I had to meet was to attend a mandatory meal planning class. I told myself it was finally time to understand correct portion, what I could and couldn't eat, and how to control my eating instead of it controlling me. The class was located at the hospital and was a smaller conference room that held twelve people. When I exited the elevator signs directed me to the conference room. There was a table in the center of the room where the nurse/instructor that worked for Bariatric Surgeons had set up a station. The chairs were lined up against the walls in a 'U' shape so that everyone had an unobstructed view.

I was one of the first to arrive and was using the same strategy as before to find an end seat close to the exit. In retrospect, it was a silly concern but it made me feel comfortable knowing I had an exit strategy if necessary. Again the usual variety of obese filtered in and it was the same routine ... small talk and a faint air of anxiety and anticipation. The nurse started by introducing herself as Shirley, the goal of the meeting and began by discussing portion sizes. I was rather relieved to see that she was no supermodel, which made me feel much more comfortable. She was in her 40's, about 5'8 and around 180 pounds. The last thing anyone needed was a Barbie doll looking down on us because we were all overweight.

    The more Shirley spoke the more I came to like her down to earth attitude, non-judgmental attitude. She certainly did a great job shocking us into the realization of what proper portion size actually entailed. She used doll-sized plastic pieces of meat and vegetables to demonstrate how much you could eat and I was reminded of those play kitchens for little girls with the miniature sized dishes and utensils. The portion sizes were about the same as the individual cereal boxes you bought in packs, and when placed on a plate, there seemed to be a lot more plate than portion. Obviously this was designed to get our attention and it certainly worked.

    Even though I enjoyed the meeting and what Shirley had to say, I didn't fully comprehend the implications of what she taught us. The portions she showed us was all you could eat. It wasn't a matter of choice to eat more if you wanted because your stomach no longer had the capacity to hold a lot of food. This wasn't about cutting back or avoiding certain foods, it was about forever changing your eating habits. At the end of the presentation there were questions and of course I didn't say a word. There was couple there and the husband was scheduled for surgery while his wife attended for support. His question struck a chord with all of us ... if you were out in the heat and drank a bottle water because you were thirsty, what would happen?

    Shirley explained that the smaller stomach couldn't hold that much water and that it would regurgitate. You would know immediately that you have over filled the pouch, but after a few times you would learn to slow down and drink smaller quantities. It really was about completely learning a new way to eat and drink. Thoroughly chewing food was also important because it had to fit in the pouch, which was small and could only hold so much food or liquid. Otherwise, any excess amount would come back up. It was very black and white. You trained yourself to eat smaller amounts and that is how weight was lost. Your body would simply prevent you from overeating and if you tried to abuse it, you would get sick. I still remember the effect of these words. This was no diet you could cheat on, and the implications were serious if you didn't follow the protocol.

Then the man asked that if drinking a bottle of water was impossible, what about a bottle of beer? Shirley explained that because beer was carbonated, it would expand the pouch. Carbonated drinks were also permanently off the list. He looked at his wife and didn't look too pleased. I couldn't help but laugh, even though the question was a valid one. I knew he was thinking if he couldn't drink half a beer, how would he manage one bottle? But it was details like this that could easily present a challenge after surgery. Surgery was the first, and in some ways, perhaps the easiest step. It was the maintenance and adherence to the lifestyle changes afterward that would present the greatest problem for people trying to adapt.

Shirley agreed that his question was quite a good one. With a smaller pouch, it would be easier to become intoxicated more quickly. The point was quite interesting to me because it never crossed my mind that beer would get into your system faster since the stomach was smaller. His wife commented that he would be a cheap date and I laughed again. It wasn't funny, but it was. I was glad that you could find humor in any situation and it made me feel better to know that we all had the same issues and concerns.

Since the meeting was concluding, Shirley introduced us to the supplements. She had several samples that were offered through the bariatric nutritional sites online but which you could buy anywhere. It was just her job to hand out samples. There was calcium, protein and multivitamins in a variety of brands and flavors for everyone to try first before buying them. She concluded the meeting by letting us pick which favors and brands we wanted while she collected the $35 payment for the class.

When I got home I told Allen about the meeting. He was pleased with my progress and proud of how everything seemed to be falling into place. After dinner we sat on the couch and looked through the supplements I had selected. I decided to test the calcium supplement first, which was in a single pack and a typical round shape. It seemed nothing out of the ordinary, but the taste was horrible and my tongue started swelling. I was alarmed because I had never suffered a reaction to a supplement before. Well, that certainly put me off trying that brand, so I went and picked up a chewable chocolate flavored chew that I thought I would be able to keep down. It was much better than the sample calcium that she had given us and now I understood why she had so many to give out, as no one liked them.

My experience with the protein shake powder was even worse. This time I was immediately sick to my stomach, and I barely drank a quarter of it. Honestly, I thought the calcium supplement was bad, but the shake was beyond disgusting. If weight loss was the goal here, it certainly worked because I couldn't imagine anyone wanting to swallow this horrible chalky stuff.

Now I was getting worried since I didn't like any of the free samples of vitamins she had given us. I kept wondering if I was going to be able to do this, considering I couldn't even handle the samples. After a few days I realized that if this was going to work I had to find a protein shake that I liked, so I managed to find a breakfast shake that contained no added sugar. It tasted like chocolate milk mixed with chalk, but it was ten times better than the sample and I could actually drink it without wanting to throw up. I preferred the pre-made shakes instead those you had to mix because they tasted better and smoother. The only downside to that was that I would have to drink six shakes a day to consume my protein requirements, as one shake contained only eleven grams of protein.

Realistically, there was no way I could drink that much of anything so I knew I had to find another protein source to satisfy my daily requirement of sixty-four grams. This is where the eggs, cheese and meat came into the picture. I liked these high protein foods and that counted toward my daily amount. I did drink three shakes a day at breakfast and as my snack and late snack. Shirley told us to eat six meals a day instead of three otherwise we wouldn't get our required nutrients if we didn't, but we were talking about Barbie sized rather than normal sized meals. I bought block cheese, cut it into pieces and filled several baggies so I could just grab one and go. I also started eating cottage cheese, which I had never tried until now. It had never appealed to me but after trying those shakes, it started tasting pretty good.

The next phase was to have an EKG at Dr. Reed's office. I didn't know what to expect because I'd never had one before, but it didn't take long and was painless. The nurse applied patches to various locations on my chest and clipped wires to it. Another $75 gone in less than an hour. I was seriously starting to consider a career in the medical field since it seemed to pay so well. Frustrated at having to pay up front for these visits, I spoke to the insurance company and they assured me they would reimburse me for most of the claims after I had the surgery. At first it didn't make sense to me, but I then I assumed they did this to ensure people went through with the surgery. At any rate, I was going to do whatever was necessary to lose weight.

The insurance company also required me to attend a group support meeting, which I wasn't happy about. The thought it was embarrassing, and I wasn't looking forward to attending another big person meeting. But it was required so I attended. I went alone because I didn't want Allen to bear the brunt of my embarrassment. The meeting was of course at an exercise/rehab facility close to the hospital. I had my quick exit strategy down pat by now so I arrived my usual few minutes early so I could see the type of people attending, Needless to say as soon I entered I found myself in a gym. I started to feel a little panicky because I thought the meeting would be held in a class or meeting room, so I asked a staff member who directed me to a meeting room down the hallway.

There were about thirty chairs inside; including extra large chairs which I was grateful I didn't need yet. People soon started arriving and they were very pleasant, ordinary looking people. Once you went down the hall there was a room that was more rectangular shaped. Two rows of chairs faced one side of the room. I of course grabbed the end chair on the far side of the room and watched as people started to come in. Like the seminar, there were people of every race, age and size, with about an equal amount of men and woman. The speaker was a woman in her mid-forties who successfully had gastric bypass surgery. She was there to tell everyone her story but unfortunately she wanted us to share our names and stories first.

I'm not sure what I was really expecting, but I found myself feeling comfortable and less anxious about the meeting. The meeting started off by everyone introducing themselves as the speaker insisted. They started from the back, but because I was seated in the middle of the group, by the time it was my turn nobody was really interested. I was fine with that because I didn't really want to talk about my situation in front of a group of strangers.

It turned out to be a mixed crowd as several people already had the surgery while others like myself had attended because it was required. Those that had the surgery were very pleased and some had lost fifty, sixty or even one-hundred pounds. No one had any negative experiences and their pride at their success and the effect weight loss had on their lives really showed, which boosted my confidence even more. The more I listened to what the others had to say, the more I realized that the surgery would be a good decision.

One patient in particular stuck in my mind. She had been sitting at the back of the room and showed us her 'before' picture along with a list of medications she was taking at the time. Her situation was truly frightening and she was well on her way to dying at an early age. She was in her fifties and had suffered from poor health, including diabetes, high blood pressure, and several other conditions. When she started speaking I wasn't sure what she was going to say because she was practically bouncing with happiness. I wasn't sure if she was high on something or if she was just high on life, but to see how much the surgery had impacted someone affected far more than anything else. Here was the confirmation I was looking for.

The woman told us she couldn't play with her grandchildren either outside or in the house because of her health, and this was a critical factor in her decision. She couldn't wait to show us her before and after pictures and she had no issues with the surgery. As a success story, she was bursting with confidence and wanted to come to the meeting and tell everyone what a great experience it was for her and that she highly recommended the surgery. Thanks to her weight loss, she was no longer diabetic, no longer was taking multiple medications, and was down to two pills a day instead of a handful. Now I truly understood the implications of how adversely obesity could affect my health and my life. The surgery had given her a second chance at a better life so she could become the person that she wanted to be. She wasn't a size ten, but she was so happy to be a healthier size that it really didn't matter what size she was. The important factor was that she could walk comfortably and get off more than half of her medications.

I listened to several other stories, some of which were funny and some were truly inspiring. I was far from alone in my situation, and I felt a sense of relief that I had options that could change my life for the better.

Then the speaker started preparing us for some of the issues we might face after surgery. Now it was time for reality to set in. Yes, there were many advantages to the procedure, but there were also the inevitable negatives. First she mentioned loose or sagging skin, vitamin deficiency and passing gas. Well, the last item took pretty much all of us by surprise. Some of the others told us about how they were passing gas more than normal. I couldn't help but laugh with everyone else because they way the explained it was hilarious. Though it was funny, the problem greatly concerned me as I didn't want to be have to deal with this. The speaker even mentioned that there were special tablets to help mask the smell of the gas. Okay ... now I was starting to worry and wondered if it was uncontrollable. No one mentioned that, but the last thing I wanted to do was go around stinking up the house or the office.

Overall, the meeting went very well and I planned to attend another one after the surgery. Everyone made me feel very comfortable with the decision that I was trying to make. They confirmed that it would be a great way for me to lose weight and get my life back on track. After the meeting the couple sitting behind me patted me on the back and reassured me that I would be fine with the surgery. A woman in the front row said that her husband didn't want her to have the surgery and wasn't happy that she was attending the meeting. The more she talked about her situation, the more we realized her husband was afraid that she would leave him when she had more confidence in herself. It wasn't an abusive relationship, but he seemed to be convinced that when she lost weight she would divorce him. I'm sure there was more to the situation than she wanted to share beyond a husband's concern about his wife having the surgery, but relationship issues were another aspect of the surgery I had never thought about.

A man that had come late to the meeting literally danced his way into the room. The speaker noticed him and introduced him as someone that had lost 150 pounds after gastric bypass surgery and was loving life. He was slim and beamed with happiness, though he did have sagging skin under his arms and in the stomach area. He told us he was almost to the point where he was considering cosmetic surgery to remove the excess skin.

An older woman told us that she regretted not having the surgery sooner. I asked her if she had to measure her portions all the time but she told me that she didn't. Your stomach told you when you had enough. I wished she had told me this before I spent $50 on a fancy electronic scale to weigh my food after the surgery, but I never would have imagined that my own stomach would do the job better than a scale. She said that it would be easy to figure out how much you could handle, and it wasn't as complicated has people thought it might be. She said your body would tell you as long as you listened to it. Then she leaned over to whisper to me that I was young enough that my skin would snap back into place. I was more than a little surprised when she mentioned that, but I just smiled and thanked her. She did have a point, and I wondered if that would happen.

That was the conclusion of the meeting and I left with a smile on my face. No one made me uncomfortable or embarrassed. As a matter of fact, I laughed and really enjoyed the meeting and I was looking forward to attending another. That was another check mark off the list. So now it was time to see what was next. During this time I was still attending weekly weigh-ins at Weight Watchers. I had to attend each week and get signed off. So I continued with my tasks in preparation for the surgery.

One day, I was reviewing my checklist to ensure everything was completed except for the diet. I noticed my weight was fluctuating. One week I lost weight and the next I gained it, but I discovered that it depended on the time of day I weighed myself. In the afternoon I always weighed more, so it seemed that I was retaining all that water I was supposed to drink throughout the day. Okay, maybe the ole pizza or burger was helping as well, because no way was I retaining all that water. I felt like an old women running to the bathroom ten times a day during work. Thankfully no one mentioned anything. Of course I had to ensure I went before I drove home because then I'd be looking to make a rather frantic pit stop en route.

***

Step by step I was getting closer to my goal. My diet was to be completed in February. All my doctors sent their records to Dr. Reed's office to prove that I had been overweight for at least five years prior to the surgery. Everything was checking out and it looked like I was going to be approved for the surgery. After getting all the information to Margaret she was able to update my file. As I attended the meeting and appointments they sent the results to Dr. Reed office to be placed in my file. Once I finished the three-month diet I faxed in the information to Dr. Reed's nurse and she completed my application to submit everything to the insurance company. After waiting two weeks for a response, the nurse called and told that I had been approved for the surgery!

It was almost like a dream. I had worked so hard getting everything together and making sure I did everything correctly, and I was proud of my achievement. I was excited to finally lose weight and not have to worry about my belly fat bulging through my shirt or worrying about finding cute clothes. I was going to be slim one day and I couldn't wait. After the seemingly endless preparation, the big day was going to March 14th.

Now came the hardest part ... telling my family about my decision. This was probably going to be the most difficult task since I knew everyone was going to have a different reaction. The first person I decided to tell was my father. I knew he would be the easiest person to tell and he would want to know honestly why I wanted to have the surgery and if it was a decision I was happy about. Once he understood that I was serious about the surgery, I knew he would support me and stand behind my decision. So I went to his mechanic's shop to break the good news.

As always, when Dad saw me drive up he grabbed a rag and started cleaning his hands as he walked toward me. He was dressed in his typical T-shirt and jeans soiled from working on cars all day. Even now he still had his thick, dark hair and had slimmed down to 150 lbs.

My parents were divorced and I was an only child so I cherished the time we spent together. I started out by asking him for his opinion on something that I had been considering for a long time. Of course I had his full attention then, so I told him that I had been thinking about having weight loss surgery.

Dad gave me that look that always told me he was concerned by lowering his head and knitting his eyebrows together. He asked how serious the surgery was and I was truthful about that it was serious surgery, but that I had also done my research and attended the meetings and appointments. Then I explained how they would cut my stomach to make a smaller pouch and reroute to the intestines. He asked how long had I been thinking about this and I told him it had been quite a while, but I emphasized that I had researched the subject exhaustively to ensure the surgery was safe for me.

Dad was always a good listener. I saw that he considered everything I said. He asked about the doctors and how I came to choose them. I replied by telling him that I'd done my homework and the team of doctors checked out and was board certified. Then he asked if this is something that I truly wanted and I told him it was. He said if that's what I wanted then to go ahead, and that he would be there for me and help anyway he could. He just wanted to make sure that I would be okay. If I was one-hundred percent certain this is what I wanted, then it would be a good idea if it would help me finally lose weight.

I told him that the insurance company would pay for it. Since I had vacation time owed from work I could take the time off without losing any pay. When dad told me to let me know when he needed to be there, I almost cried from relief. It was such a weight off my shoulders because I knew if he didn't like the idea of surgery then my mother wouldn't be happy at all. Now at least I had the support of someone else beyond Allen. I waited a few more days to tell anyone else.

My sister-in-law Marie was the next person I told. She had called to see if she could spend some time with Sam, so on Sunday Allen and I dropped him off for a few hours. As soon as we pulled into the driveway she came out to greet us with hugs and kisses for Sam before he even got out of the car. She truly was the best sister-in-law I could ask for, and although she was a gorgeous brunette that could pass for a model and took the best possible care of herself, she was in no way conceited or looked down on me in anyway. I didn't tell her the same way I told my father. Marie was a worrier and because she was Allen's older sister, she tended to play the loving mother hen quite a bit.

I took a different approach with her and mentioned that I'd been doing a lot of research and since I wasn't able to get pregnant, I talked to my doctors and they highly suggested that weight loss surgery would be great for me. I told her about all the steps I had successfully completed and that I had been approved for the surgery. She seemed comfortable with the idea that doctors had suggested it. Allen assured her that this was something that I had been considering for quite a while and was something I really wanted to do for myself and my family.

Marie had the usual questions and concerns about the surgery and recovery time. She asked about taking time off for work and how I would handle eating afterward. By now I knew how to answer all her questions and when she asked if I really felt surgery was the answer for my weight loss, I assured her that it was going to be fine and that I had done all my homework. She was very surprised but I think she wanted to do some of her own research too. She seemed okay with my decision but knowing her, she would be on the computer Googling everything she could to ensure I was aware of the complications and advantages of the surgery.

As for my mother, I decided to wait until the surgery date drew closer before telling her because I didn't want to worry her. Unlike my father, she wouldn't be as easy to convince that having major surgery was an answer to weight loss, and I wasn't quite ready to deal with her concerns just yet.

Chapter 5 - New Beginnings

I was sitting at the kitchen table looking at my planner and had calculated that I would be off work for approximately three weeks. Admittedly I was anxious about telling my boss since it wasn't the best time to be away from the office. The economy wasn't doing well and people were being laid off from their jobs all around the surrounding counties. I had also been recently promoted to the lead position because Amelia and Leah both had decided to be stay-at-home moms. While I was able to find a replacement for Leah, I was still interviewing for Amelia's replacement.

While going through my calendar I also realized that I hadn't had my period in several weeks. It was almost like an afterthought since after so many years of trying unsuccessfully to have a baby I didn't even consider the possibility that I might actually be pregnant. I'd always had a fairly regular cycle, and because my symptoms generally warned me when my period was due, I never really bothered keeping track of actual dates beyond those that corresponded with holidays or special events.

Still, I had to make sure before I could proceed with the bypass surgery, so I decided to get a pregnancy test kit. I had gotten a false negative with Sam, so I didn't really trust the accuracy of the tests, but after already spending so much on out of pocket medical expenses, I chose to buy a kit from the dollar store. I didn't want to have a waste a visit to the doctor only to be told I wasn't pregnant.

As far as I was concerned this was simply another item on my check list to deal with. I went to the local dollar store to purchase a double kit, but interestingly it took forever to find the test kits because for some reason they were kept behind the counter. So now pregnancy test kits were treated like cigarettes? Fortunately I didn't have to provide any identification to buy the kit, or that really would have been ridiculous. I hadn't yet told Allen about it because I didn't want to raise his hopes that I might be pregnant, especially since I was planning on having the surgery. In maybe two or three years I would consider it, but not now.

Or so I thought ... after the first test, I was shocked speechless to find a positive. But how could that be possible after trying unsuccessfully to have a baby for three years? I decided to take the other test and sure enough, it was also a positive. Then I thought because I was using a cheap dollar store test kit the results were probably unreliable, but I had followed the instructions. I couldn't believe it. Like the proverbial 'deer caught in the headlights', I just stood in the bathroom leaning against the counter staring at the test.

The bathroom had three large windows so there was plenty of light. For the longest time I couldn't do anything but look at the results. All of us had prayed for another baby for so long ... was this really possible? It was such a shock to me. The thought had never crossed my mind that I would get pregnant. This was one of the reasons I wanted to have the surgery is so that I could get pregnant and suddenly I'm pregnant without even having the surgery. I felt fine, and hadn't suffered any nausea or symptoms typical of early stage pregnancy.

I really needed Allen to see the results so I knew it wasn't just my imagination. I wanted to feel excited, but I was also cautious because I didn't want to be disappointed either. All I could really focus on was the irony of the timing. Well, we really wanted a baby so now our prayers were finally answered.

Allen was out fishing behind the house so I drove out to show him what was going on. When I got there he was in the aluminum boat in the middle of the pond. It really was a lovely rural setting, green, lush and full of trees and the serenade of birdsong. Though we had about an acre of land, a hunting club abutted our property line, and Allen had leased the land for hunting and fishing since it was so close to the house, which gave us access to hundreds of acres and several fishing ponds.

Since Allen often fished at different ponds, he always let me know where he was so I could find him in case of an emergency or I needed to reach for him any reason. This was a standard buddy system for hunters during hunting season in case someone was injured or unconscious and couldn't call for help. They also tended to keep their phones on silent and didn't always check for messages. If a hunter needed help they would remain in the same location until someone came looking for them. This way I knew that if Allen wasn't home by reasonable amount of time after dark, I would know where to find him rather than searching hundreds of acres.

Regardless, this was one of those occasions when I needed to see him so he could witness my concern/joy/surprise/shock. I knew where he was by the distance, so I drove the quarter mile to the access point and followed the trails out to the pond.

When Allen noticed me drive up he immediately realized something was wrong because I rarely drove to the ponds. We'd gone together on a number of occasions just to enjoy the land, but it wasn't a place I'd go alone and because it was private land, we rarely saw anyone else. Allen immediately started the trolling motor and steered the boat toward the shore. I noticed him watching my face to gauge my expression, but I didn't look upset, just a little concerned.

Allen called out to me asking what was wrong as the boat approached, but I didn't want to shout out that I might be pregnant, so I just yelled back that it was nothing serious. Once he came ashore, he asked what was wrong and I told him that I had taken a pregnancy test because I had missed my period. He was frankly stunned, since we had been trying for so long and nothing had happened. The irony of the timing also didn't escape him. I asked him to confirm if I was reading the results correctly. By now my heart was racing as I watched him carefully check the results, which both read positive. He couldn't believe it either, but he had a little smirk on his face that turned into a smile when he confirmed the readings were positive. Then he advised me to check with Dr. Jones to make sure before I got my hopes up. For a moment all we could do was look at each other as neither of us could believe it. Why would I get pregnant now?

Since it was Sunday, I had to wait until the next day before I could call Dr. Jones' office. I asked for his nurse, Lisa. I knew that Lisa would recognize my name and I told her that I needed to make an appointment as soon as possible because I thought I might be pregnant. I was worried because I had been approved for my surgery, and now I was torn between having my wish for a child granted but also not wanting to waste the time, money and effort I had put into getting approved. I was more than excited and deeply grateful to be pregnant, but I was also committed to changing my life and health and the surgery was the means to accomplish that goal.

Fortunately Dr. Jones saw me the same day and I took a pregnancy test. The waiting was agonizing, and I could only wonder if this was a sign from God that I shouldn't have the surgery? Where things were better left alone? Then I thought about the positive changes the surgery would bring to not only my life, but for my family as well if I were fitter and healthier. When Lisa finally called me into a room, I only had to wait a few minutes before Dr. Jones came in with a big smile on my face. I remember his words so well as he congratulated me ... I was going to have a baby!

To say I was overwhelmed by the results was an understatement. I still couldn't believe that after three years of struggling to conceive and spending not only hard-earned money but months of time, not to mention finally getting approved by the insurance company, I now found myself pregnant. I should have been elated, but all I could think about was what would happen to my surgery and everything I invested into it. The more I thought about possibly having to start the protracted approval process all over again, the more emotional and confused I became. Perhaps because I was no longer focusing on becoming pregnant my body finally allowed it to happen.

I was delighted to be pregnant, but not with the timing. I called Allen as soon as I left the office. He was excited and concerned at the same time. We both wanted another baby but neither of knew what was going to happened with the surgery. As I returned to the car the reality that I was finally pregnant finally started to sink. By the time I got to the car I was practically skipping with joy! Since I hadn't told many people about the surgery I didn't have much explaining to do when I called everyone to tell them the great news. Mom still didn't know about the surgery as I had put off telling her until closer to date. She was the next person I called and she was so excited about the news. She loves kids, especially grandchildren, but just not too many, of course. Dad and Marie were both overjoyed as well.

As everything started settling and we had gotten used to the news of my pregnancy, I called Dr. Reed's office and told them that I had just found out I was pregnant after being approved for the surgery. I asked if I would lose everything I had worked so hard for, but the coordinator told me that I had up to a year to have the surgery after approval. After that, I would have to start over, but after nine months of pregnancy and six weeks of recovery, I realized that would still leave me with a cushion of almost two months to have the surgery. If I scheduled the surgery six weeks after having the baby, everything could still work out.

When I went to see Dr. Jones, I was eager to hear what he had to say. I was so worried I might go over-term because I was induced with Sam, so I was concerned it would be the same with my second child. Dr. Jones suggested that six weeks after having a c-section would work well for the surgery, which is what I had hoped he would say. I was so relieved I almost felt like crying, since now this meant I could have the both a baby and the surgery and all my effort wouldn't be in vain. I certainly didn't want to start the process over and was happy that the worry was over, but now I had to make sure I could schedule the surgery in that two month period. Since the surgery would be well into the future, it might actually be an advantage since all the people ahead of me at the seminar would have signed up sooner.

I was thinking November or December, so I called Dr. Reed's office and discussed the date with the coordinator. She was able to schedule me for November 7th, which would be perfect. I would have six to eight weeks of maternity leave followed by two to three weeks of short term disability.

Since I had been taking quite a few long lunches my co-workers were starting to suspect something was going on. I assured them that I wasn't looking for another job and at that point I realized it was time to tell everyone that I was preparing to have weight loss surgery. This was the most difficult part for me as I considered it a private matter and I really didn't want to hear anyone's smart ass comments or snide remarks. I remember returning from lunch one afternoon. We had a sign-in sheet on the counter at reception to let other employees know when we would return if someone was looking for us. I had picked up a cheeseburger combo from a local restaurant on my way back from shopping, and when I set the bag on the counter to sign in, my boss said, "Well, that's not healthy for you." I remember thinking that it wasn't, but if she would have said anything else, if wouldn't have been healthy for her either.

Those were the thoughtless and hurtful comments that I wanted to avoid, but of course people were going to be people. There's always going to be someone skinny ready to say, "If you would just put down the cookie then you'll be fine." Well, it just doesn't work that way. Besides my co-workers, I also told two close friends at work. Julie and Elaine were my support group if someone said or did something to upset me. Almost everyone was positive and many were curious about the surgery, how it worked and what happened afterward. I decided that I would just be honest. If anyone asked I would tell them. I figured I had two choices, either be open about it or have people talk about it behind my back, so I chose to talk about the surgery. Discussing my personal struggles with my weight was one of the most difficult things for me to do.

Of course news spread even more rapidly at work that I was pregnant. If anyone was the subject of office gossip, it was certainly me as I felt everyone with the possible exception of the cleaning crew was talking about it. When I walked into the break room someone would congratulate me on the baby and then ask about the surgery, so at times it was almost overwhelming. Still, I had set the wheels in motion, and the interest in my progress might help me stay on track later on.

***

Thirty-eight weeks into term I had only gained nine pounds. I felt good and was proud that I did such a great job controlling my weight during the pregnancy, as I gained the same amount that I did with Sam. As my due date approached, Dr. Jones confirmed that I would be having a c-section. This was great news and would allow me to plan my surgery. Now I could provide Dr. Reed's coordinator an estimated date that Dr. Jones would release me so that she could schedule the surgery date.

Finally my due date of September 18th arrived and I was admitted to the hospital for my c-section. The procedure went well and I had my son, Chase. He was perfect, handsome and healthy. We were so proud of our new addition to the family. Chase had minor blood sugar problems that keep him in the NICU for a few days, but Sam also and the same issue so we weren't concerned because we already knew the process. After everything was straightened out we were able to bring him home.

Eight weeks after Chase was born, which was the allocated period for c-section maternity leave, I started reviewing my surgery information again since there was a two-week preparation period before the surgery. Feeling a sense of excitement about how things were turning out in my life, I stayed in constant contact with Dr. Reed office to make sure all the arrangements were made, including confirmation of my surgery date on November 10. The thought of a new, slim me motivated the hell out of me, and I began to fantasize about shopping for cute clothes in a smaller size. I imagined going out with friends and family without worrying about how I looked or whether my rolls of fat were showing. Even better, I pictured myself in a cute bathing suit and swimming without worrying about what everyone else thought. Look out world, the new Ellie was coming soon!

Part of my preparation for surgery was taking vitamins before the surgery that included multivitamins, sub-lingual B-12, and calcium. Dr. Reed would give me two prescriptions before leaving the hospital. There was also a two week diet prior to surgery. Once again I thought that if I could have stuck to a proper diet in the first place I wouldn't be in this situation. When I attended the pre-surgery support group meeting Shirley told us that it was critical to follow the diet, because it reduced the size of the liver and allowed the surgeon to maneuver around easier. She also warned us that the surgeon would know if you didn't follow the diet correctly because there would be white spots on the liver and it would be slippery or greasy. This made the liver more difficult to handle. Needless to say that elicited quite an image in my mind about what mine must have looked like and it probably wasn't good. I've tried so many times to stick to a diet, but when budget was an issue and there were only certain items in the refrigerator, you ate what was there.

By now almost everyone knew about the surgery, but I had also decided to mention it to my friend, Beth. We'd been friends since the sixth grade, but even though we didn't see each other as much as we used to, we still kept in touch. I was surprised that she wasn't too keen on my decision even though her mother had gastric bypass surgery when we were in school. At the time I knew that she had the procedure, but didn't actually know what it was. Beth told me not to tell anyone. I just thought her mom had stomach problems and was embarrassed about it. It was a new procedure back then so not many people even knew what it was.

Needless to say I was surprised when Beth told me that God made my body the way it is, and that I shouldn't mess with it by rerouting my intestines. Yet to my knowledge her mother never had any complications. She lost weight but gained it back years later after she divorced Beth's step-dad. I just thought she gained weight from the stress. Nevertheless, I considered Beth's response and told her I'd keep her updated about the surgery. Her comment was something that I took seriously, so I researched the statistics for people suffering digestive problems after surgery. Though there wasn't much information available, I assumed if there were concerns Dr. Reed would have mentioned it.

It was finally time to tell my mother, and I was feeling more than anxious because I didn't know how she would respond. It could go two ways. She would either love or hate the idea, but it was my decision and I would have to deal with whatever her reaction might be. I knew she loved me and my family with all her heart, but when it came to medical issues she was a stickler for everything being by a doctor's recommendation or else she couldn't accept it. Still, I had all the medical support I needed and I realized that ultimately I was a grown woman who had to make a decision on my own. Yes, I had asked for opinions and had carefully weighed them, but at the end of the day it was my health and my life, and I wanted to be the best I could for myself and my family.

A visit to my maternal grandmother gave me the opportunity as I knew my mother would be there. I was so nervous that my stomach was in knots, as though I was a child fixing to get a spanking after church for misbehaving during the service. Silly, I know. I was an adult and simply needed to act like one. The visit started like it always did. We chatted for a while and caught up on all the gossip, but when my grandmother went to the kitchen to finish preparing lunch, I told my mother as casually as I could that I had spoken to Dr. Jones about having weight loss surgery. Since he was also her doctor that made it easier for me to convince her that I could trust what the doctors said.

Of course she was concerned and asked me what I meant, so I explained that both Dr. Jones and Dr. Powell had suggested it. After months of research, preparation and testing, the insurance company had approved the surgery and I had already scheduled the time off work. I would combine my eight weeks of maternity leave with an additional three weeks off with short term disability. The extra time off wouldn't be that noticeable either because most people knew I would be on maternity leave. When Dr. Jones released me from his care, Dr. Reed would transfer me under his care for surgery so everything would continue smoothly.

Mom wanted to know about the surgery and asked the same questions everyone else had, so I took my time and detailed everything. Though she was initially concerned, she could see that I had thoroughly done my research and she seemed especially pleased that both my doctors had not only recommended the surgery, but were excited about it.

Then she asked what Allen thought, and I assured her that he had supported me every step of the way and was happy about my decision.

She didn't overreact in any way but took time to consider what I told her, and I saw much of myself in her quiet, private, and very independent personality. Her only concern was that I had taken all necessary precautions to ensure everything went well. If I was okay with everything, then she was as well.

The relief I felt from knowing I had her approval was indescribable. She was going to stand behind me on my decision and wasn't going to try and talk me out of it. Knowing that I had the support of my entire family and that they stood behind me was really a turning point for me. I no longer had to worry about anyone else's opinion because it was just an opinion.

I also told my grandmother later that day after my mother left. Like Beth, she didn't care for the idea. She didn't want me taking chances with surgery just to lose weight, though she agreed I needed to lose weight. In her opinion, I should have exhausted all my options before considering something as drastic as surgery. Her opinion really made me think about it some more, but after weighing the pros and cons, I still felt gastric bypass surgery was the best choice for me.

***

I had a schedule appointment with pre-admissions before surgery and I was excited about going. The pre-admission was for blood work, an EKG, and to complete paperwork. My mother and Chase came with me to keep me company in the event the process took a while, but the pre-admission was easier than I expected. Ten minutes after I signed in a staff member asked me medical questions and told me that the copayment was due on the day of my surgery. Once I had completed the medical paperwork, I had my blood work and EKG done quite quickly as the staff were fast and professional. My results came back fine about ten minutes later. They did a follow up EKG just to ensure nothing had changed since the previous test results.

The last step of pre-admissions was talking to a nurse about what to expect and prepare for, as well as fill out more paperwork. It was like a mini-exam because we covered the same questions a doctor would ask. Though I was concerned about taking anti-depressants, it seemed to have no bearing on my surgery. I was impressed that the nurse listened to my concerns and emphasized that I would be taken care of. Her questions were beyond routine, I could see that she wanted to assure me about the surgery and I felt less anxious after speaking with her. When I was finished, I returned to the waiting room to find several smiling women admiring Chase. I left feeling more than positive about my decision to have the surgery. I wasn't scared or nervous. In fact, I felt good. I knew that my life was about to take a new direction and I was excited to get started.

***

  The big day was approaching fast, so I made sure everything was ready and organized. Sam was in elementary school by now so he would stay with Marie, with my niece Courtney watching him after school until Marie got home from work. Sam knew I was having surgery but didn't fully understand what was going on, so we explained that it would be the same as when I had Chase. He was comfortable with that so we didn't give him any further details. Chase would stay with my cousin Sandy at my grandmothers house, and since everyone lived within a short distance of each other, it would be convenient for everyone, not to mention exciting as everyone was looking forward to babysitting.
  I would only be staying overnight and would be up and walking soon after surgery so I packed comfortable clothes. The last thing I wanted was to be flashing as I walked down the hall. But nothing compared to that nasty stuff I had to drink the day before surgery. Disgusting didn't even begin to describe it. It wasn't medicine awful, but sweet tasting awful. It was ten times worse than the most sugary soda and I initially thought I could just gulp it down, but that nauseating cherry flavor seemed to get stuck in my throat. I even made sure it was really cold because I had read somewhere that it went down better that way, but it made no difference. Fortunately there was no time limit to drink it, as it took me about three hours to get it down without gagging. I did have to go to the bathroom several times, but nothing like I had imagined it would be.

Finally, it was time to go. Everything was ready, so Allen and I got up early enough on the Tuesday morning to make the forty-five minute drive to the hospital without rushing as I had to be there at 5:00 am. The house was clean and there was food in the fridge because I knew I wouldn't be able to do much for a little while. On the drive to the hospital, I started thinking about the surgery. While I imagine most people would have been anxious or nervous, I was pretty confident that everything would be fine.

Allen and I were both quiet, partially because it was 4:00 a.m., but also because we were both lost in our thoughts. It was raining, and still dark. We traveled the interstate, which was the most direct route and not particularly scenic beyond the trees that were barely visible in the pre-dawn twilight. Normally we might have bickered about the route since I had my shortcuts to Atlanta, but today, the route wasn't important. A successful surgery without complications was the most important thing right now. Allen asked if I was really ready to go ahead with the surgery and I reassured him that I was. If I wanted to change my mind for any reason he wouldn't hesitate to turn back and go home. I thanked him for his support and knew that he would be there for me. At this point I was confident because I knew in my heart that I had done all the research possible. I also knew that the surgery wasn't just for me, but for my family.

Inevitably it crossed my mind that I might not see my family again. I did tear up a little when I thought of the possibility of Allen raising our kids without me, but I knew in my heart that if something did go wrong that he would take good care of them. Of course they would miss their mother, but Allen was a wonderful father and would love them enough for both of us. I wanted to tell Allen to make sure that if something did happen to let them know that I loved them with all my heart today and forever. Perhaps I should have talked to Allen about this, but I didn't want to frighten him with that possibility, nor did I want to start feeling anxious by seeing his reaction.

I don't know if Allen was driving fast or I was simply preoccupied, but before I knew it we were pulling up to the entrance of Medical Center. It was still raining so I quickly ducked inside. I was quite familiar with the facility because it was where I had attended my first seminar, had my various doctors' visits and numerous tests. There would be necessary preparations before the surgery so I knew it would still be awhile before I was ready to go. While Allen parked the car, I walked through the sliding glass double doors into a waiting area with booths labeled A, B, C for patient registration.

There was only one couple in waiting area when we arrived. They were already seated in the two chairs closest to the registration desk. It was a large, rectangular area with about twenty-five chairs in rows lining the walls. Because it was so early, there was only one administrator at the booth. The man wearing jogging pants had to be the one having surgery out of the two of them. I had worn jeans and a T-shirt so I could be comfortable. I signed my name and found two seats for myself and Allen far enough away from the couple to give us enough space between us so that we could all talk without overhearing each other's conversations. Allen had arrived by then and sat beside me, though we really didn't say much since we were probably a little nervous and lost again in our thoughts about what was going to happen.

After about fifteen minutes, the female administrator at Booth A called out the man's name and he provided them his information, insurance card and copayment. During that time several other staff members started arriving with their lunch bags and umbrellas. I watched as they passed us and entered a door marked 'staff only'.

After the man returned to his seat, the administrator called my name so she could get my information too. When I sat at the booth she asked for my insurance card, driver's license and the $250 copayment. After entering my information, she scanned my cards and printed several documents to open a file. One of the printouts contained the information for the wristband that she placed on my arm. At that point she told me to have a seat until someone called my name. I had to admit I still wasn't anxious but rather more curious about what would happen next. I smiled at Allen as I returned to my seat, and he gave me a kiss and a hug. He asked if everything was okay and I told him I would be called soon.

Almost immediately a nurse in blue scrubs walked through the double doors and called my name. Allen and I looked at each other and got up to follow her through a series of hallways and turns leading to a room where two nurses waited for me. Debbie was the head nurse and stood beside a hospital bed at the table making sure she had everything she needed. The second nurse, Eadie, checked everything on the tables, which were very organized. Debbie was in her forties, about 5'8 and around 200 pounds with short, no-nonsense brown hair streaked with gray. Eadie was a few years younger, of average size and weight, with shoulder-length brown wavy hair.

They both wore white scrubs, unlike other staff I had seen in blue scrubs. I don't know why I noticed the colors, but it was one of those minor details you tended to pick up on for some reason. The hospital had that early morning feel because the halls were very quiet and we walked past several rooms clean and ready for patients. They were painted in cheerful light colors.

Debbie led me into the last room on the right. She handed me the gown folded on the bed along with a plastic bag and showed me a bathroom where I could change. I noticed that the blue gown bearing the hospital logo was made for larger people, which was a relief. While I changed, Allen waited in a chair by the window. Though it was still dark, the first blush of dawn touched the sky. As I changed, I realized that Sam and Chase were probably still asleep and wouldn't even know what was happening, which was fine. I was excited about it, I was looking forward to what was going to happen next. Even though it was a hospital and preparing for surgery, I felt like I was being pampered. The staff was dedicated to ensure I was okay and comfortable. In a way, it was actually nice to feel special. Everyone was there for me and I was the center of attention. I felt at ease and as strange as it may have sounded, I was almost enjoying the experience.

After I changed into the gown, I placed my clothes into a bag Debbie provided. I returned to the room, handed the bag to Allen and sat in the bed. Debbie was smiling and very cheerful. She made me feel very comfortable, and her attitude helped me relax and feel confident. I was smiling, a little nervous and excited at the same time. She explained that she was going get me prepped for surgery. Eadie left and I never saw her again. The process was very quick, and by now the sun was rising. The sky was washed with a vivid palette of orange and yellow, and I noticed a pleasant tree-shaded patio on a nearby rooftop where people could enjoy the fresh air without leaving the hospital.

As Debbie finished up an orderly in scrubs walked in and asked if we were ready to go. Debbie said yes and he clapped his hands and said that was great. I was struck again by how upbeat the medical staff were, which certainly helped put me at ease. Allen followed us into the hall, and as I gazed up at the ceiling light and tiles, I felt like I was in a movie scene. I felt comfortable and still wasn't that nervous.

The orderly approached a waiting area for family members that displayed monitors much like those at airports showing the progress of each patient. He told Allen that the wait would be about ninety minutes. Oddly, I realized that I had never asked how long the surgery would actually take. It never crossed my mind that Allen would have to wait that long. As my bed rolled to a stop I saw my father and his mother waiting to see me. I was so pleased they had come. Dad and Maw hugged me and kissed my cheek and told me that they loved me, while Allen leaned over that gave me a bear hug. He told me that he loved me and that he would see me in a few hours. Debbie suggested that everyone could either wait or go get some breakfast to pass the time.

While Debbie stayed with my family, the orderly wheeled into what I called the 'holding tank' for surgery. Shaped like a 'T', it consisted of sectioned off slots divided by curtains. Four sections faced each, with two at the end of the room. You could see the patient across from you but not beside you. I noticed an older man across from me who looked very concerned. He didn't appear pleased to be there, though I didn't know if he was simply nervous or just didn't want to be laying in a hospital bed in a room full of strangers. I tried to figure out why he was there. Considering his age, perhaps he was having heart surgery.

The nurse's station was in the center of the holding tank only a few feet from my bed. It was bustling, with doctors and nurses in scrubs walking around with patient files and applying arm bands. Another nurse, Sarah, approached asked if I still had my contacts in and I told her I was. She was in her mid-twenties and had a small frame with straight, shoulder length brown hair. I was struck how friendly and pleasant the nurses were. Sarah was also quite upbeat and I felt quite comfortable with her as well. I asked her if could leave my contacts in as long as possible because I couldn't see anything without them. She said it was fine as long as I didn't forget to remove them before I went in for surgery.

Dennis, a male nurse, came to set me up with my IV. Dark-haired, quite tall, and also in his twenties, he didn't instill the same confidence as the other nurses. He appeared nervous when he tried to insert the IV into my left arm, so he decided to place it in my left hand instead. It still wasn't inserted properly as it sat right where my wrist bent, but I assumed if it was an issue Sarah would have mentioned something. I didn't know if Dennis was new or just recently trained, but I didn't think it was appropriate that patients prepped for surgery had to deal with someone so obviously nervous.

While Dennis dealt with the IV, Sarah rubbed my right hand to reassure me. I asked her if Allen could come back and wait with me, so she asked Kathy, the head nurse, if that was possible. Kathy was about 5'8, of average weight with gray-peppered brown hair. I could tell by her demeanor that she was a no-nonsense type. Perched on the edge of her chair at the nurse's station, she was completely focused on her work. When Sarah returned a moment later, she explained that it wasn't allowed because it was better that family members didn't see their loved ones put to sleep. It made sense, really, as I imagined Allen wouldn't want to watch something like that. At that point I did become a little emotional, and I shed a few tears. I wasn't feeling panicky or hysterical, it was more of a scared of the unknown kind of feeling that I was sure anyone facing surgery felt.

After about ten minutes I heard a child crying. It sounded like a little girl and I could hear her parents trying to reassure her. I asked Sarah if everything was okay and she explained that the little girl was there to have her tonsils removed and was very scared. I was happy that they at least allowed the parents to come back and comfort the little girl because she really sounded frightened. It's certainly what I would have done with my own children. Thankfully they must have taken her in for surgery because then it became quiet. I assumed she must have been in a nearby bed because the older man across from me was looking toward her. At least the little girl provided a distraction to relieve my concerns, as I was feeling for the parents and how upsetting it would have been to hear her crying.

As I settled back to wait, I couldn't believe how busy it was. It almost reminded me of an airport terminal with all the doctors and nurses rushing around. Sarah asked me if it was my first surgery and I told her that I'd had a cyst removed from my fallopian tubes, though I didn't remember anything like this. I also mentioned that I'd had two c-sections. She noticed in my chart that I had recently had a baby and she asked a few questions about Chase that helped distract me. Then she asked what I did for a living and the usual questions to keep my mind occupied.

The waiting seemed to take forever but it was actually only about fifteen or twenty minutes before, Dr. Thompson, one of the doctors performing my surgery, came by to shake my hand and introduce himself. He was tall, distinguished, and with his salt and pepper hair, looked very much a typical soap opera doctor. He wore scrubs and looked prepped for surgery. I had never seen him before, but he told me he was assisting Dr. Reed. After shaking his hand, I asked him to make sure that Dr. Reed was performing the surgery as I didn't want to get mixed up with anyone else in that room. He smiled and assured me that Dr. Reed was definitely the doctor performing my gastric bypass surgery. That made me feel better, since I didn't want to be one of those people who went in for one procedure and ended up having something completely different done. That would have been beyond nightmarish.

Finally, it was time to remove my contacts. Since I had new ones in my overnight bag, I told Sarah to discard them. I took a deep breath as Sarah told me it was time for the surgery. Some operating room staff came and wheeled me through some double doors. I remember how cold the air felt on my face, though Sarah had given me a warm blanket. I absolutely loved the cozy feel and snuggled beneath it. I didn't really look at anyone in the other beds as we maneuvered out of the holding tank.

The operating room was just beyond the doors. White and sterile, I squinted against the bright overhead lights. Dr. Reed and his team waited by the operating table. I caught the gleam of instruments, but by now I was sleepy from the medication Dennis must have administered in the IV, and my eyes slowly closed. My new future was moments away ... and I hoped it would be a good one.

Chapter 6 - Success

Of course Allen and Dad had been constantly watching the monitors in the waiting room regarding my progress, but they were still anxiously waiting for one of the doctors to come out and update them. I don't remember returning to my room, though Dad held my hand assuring me that he was there by my side. Allen was brushing my hair from my face trying to wake me up.

When I tried to speak my mouth was extremely dry. Groggily, I smiled and asked Allen if I could have something, so he told Cindy, my nurse. She mentioned that I could have ice chips, but no more than a medicine cup full at a time, so she brought some. I had a couple and went back to sleep. I still wasn't in any pain, which surprised me since I had expected a considerable amount of abdominal discomfort, but I was overwhelmingly tired and wanted to sleep until the anesthesia finally wore off enough so that I could finally stay awake.

Finally, I was alert enough to chat with Allen and Dad, but I didn't want to attempt sitting up yet because I felt soreness in my abdominal area and didn't want to cause more pain by moving around. Also I knew I was on pain medication so that would be dulling any discomfort for now.

After I dozed off for a little while I felt like the anesthetic had finally worn off so I remember closing my eyes against the glare of the lights ... then suddenly I awoke in my room with Allen and Dad sitting beside me. Sunlight beamed through the window, and as my eyes focused, I found myself in a room not so different to the room where I was before the surgery. Sunlight filtered through windows framed by multicolor patterned curtains, and there was a flat screen TV mounted on the wall with a bathroom to my left.

Allen and Dad stood smiling on either side of the bed and smothered me in kisses. When they asked how I was I told them I felt drowsy but not in any pain, but all I really wanted to do at that point was go back to sleep. Allen told me that Dr. Reed had spoken with them and that the surgery had been a complete success, though the entire process from preparation, to recovery and finally returning me to my room had taken several hours, primarily because I hadn't woken up easily after the surgery. It hadn't been from any complications, but from what must have been fatigue on my part.

I called to check on my sons and let them know that I loved them and that I would be home soon.

Mom also came to see me after leaving work early. She was delighted everything had gone so well and gave me a big hug. Though she and Dad had been divorced since I was a child, they had always remained friends and had a good relationship. Dad even continued to service Mom's car, so I was happy that we are able to spend some time together.

Dad told me he would pick up the boys and bring them to spend some time with me. Though I was feeling better I was uncomfortable with the catheter. I didn't like the idea of the bag visible at the end of the bed, which I found awkward with so many visitors. Since I was able to get up and go to the bathroom, I asked Cindy if it could be removed and she told me that it was up to the doctor, because it was usually left it in until the next day. At least I was able to sit in the chair for a few minutes, but it wasn't comfortable so I got back in bed, which I found easier even though I experienced some discomfort in my stomach area. The biggest issue was that I could feel the catheter, which limited my movement.

Since Dr. Reed wanted me up and moving as soon as I felt up to it, I felt the catheter was hindering me and I really wanted it removed.

When the Dr. Reed came in to check on me he said that I was doing very well. The incisions looked great, but it was important to keep them clean. He also told me that I needed to get up and start walking down the corridor. When he mentioned that the catheter could be removed I was excited because I knew I would be fine after that. Apart from cautioning me not to overdo it, he had no other concerns and said he would be back tomorrow to check on me. It was funny to think how excited I was to have the catheter removed, but once that was out, Allen suggested we go for a walk, which was fine as I didn't want to be confined to a bed any longer than necessary. He helped me with the IV machine and heart monitor while we walked along three corridors twice. Walking was easier than I expected and I was surprised by how good I felt, though I wasn't sure if the pain medication was a factor. Regardless, it was great to be up and moving.

As I walked, I had to wonder how amazing the mind was. I had conjured up all kinds of dark scenarios where I imagined I'd be bedridden in terrible pain, but it was nothing at all like that and I knew that I had made the right decision about having the surgery. We walked down the hallways and around the nurses' station which was octagon shaped so the nurses could see every hall. It was quite busy, filled with flowers and doctors and nurses entering information onto computers and dealing with phone calls and paperwork. Allen continually asked me if I was up to making another round, but I assured him I was up to it. The purpose was to move around, not speed walk, and even with my slow progress I felt like I did a great job.

When I returned to my room, Cindy brought me lunch consisting of unsweetened tea and sugar free jello. The cherry jello was fine, but I could barely drink the tea as I hated it without sugar. I only ate about three-quarters of the jello, but Cindy assured me that I didn't need to eat more than that because my pouch was the size of a walnut at this point. I continued to chew on ice every fifteen minutes, and between walking and visiting with Dad and the boys, time passed and it was time for dinner.

I was so excited to see the boys. Dad had gone to get them and was back before I knew it. It was wonderful to see them and I felt blessed to have such a wonderful family. Sam figured out where and how to get free drinks and ice so he was starting to get restless. After giving them lots of kisses, Dad took them home so I could rest. Once again, Cindy brought more unsweetened tea, a sugar free popsicle and jello. The popsicle was tasty, but the tea was a chore to swallow. Now would come the real test as I had no choice but to carefully control what I ate.

That night I rested as much as I could while the nurses came periodically to check my vitals. By then I was beginning to feel some discomfort in my lower back, which surprised me since I had expected to feel abdominal pain. But when I informed the nurse about it she told me it was not unusual and gave me some pain medication. Later, a young technician came into my room to check on me, as he said the heart monitor didn't seem to be working properly, but it was only a technical glitch that he took care of.

***

The next morning, I was feeling pretty good other than some lower back discomfort. I got up and went to the bathroom to brush my teeth and my hair before walking up and down the corridor a few times. Dr. Reed came to check on me and gave me the good news that everything looked great and that he would discharge me today. I was so excited and couldn't wait to go home and see my boys and take it easy in the recliner, not to mention how much more comfortable Allen would be on the couch instead of a hospital recliner.

Breakfast consisted of grits and juice. I was able to eat and drink a little of both, but couldn't finish it. It was a lesson in learning that I didn't have to eat everything on my plate. My mother never instilled that habit in me, but as I got older I got into the habit of cleaning my plate because of habit and economical necessity. Now it wasn't a choice. Allen and I got ready, a nurse came in with the discharge papers, and after completing them I was free to go home. I was somewhat embarrassed that I had to be taken to the car in a larger wheelchair, but I assumed it was standard for patients like myself, and it seemed that I was the only one that even noticed.

On the way home we stopped by my grandmothers house to pick up the boys. Once again I smothered them in hugs and kisses. After visiting for a short time, we went on home to relax. The drive was quiet; I was simply enjoying the fact that the surgery was over and that I could relax. I had already purchased multi-vitamins and sugar free popsicles so I had everything I needed. After settling down with kids and getting unpacked, I settled onto the recliner and finally breathed a grateful sigh of relief mixed in with more than a little pride. I had done it … all the preparation and legwork had paid off big time! Now I felt more than ready to face the challenges that I knew would come, but at least now I felt confident that I could deal with them.

***

That night I took a shower and studied my abdomen. I had six small incisions that seemed to be taped rather than stitched or stapled. There was some bruising around the incisions but nothing unexpected considering I'd had surgery. When the nurse helped me with the discharge papers, she told me that I could take a shower but to leave the tape on until they fell off by themselves. If they hadn't fallen off after three days, I could remove them in the shower. Standing under the warm water was so refreshing and I felt really relaxed afterward. I took my time with everything I did and avoided lifting anything heavier than Chase, who weighed only eight pounds.

Two of my friends called and wanted to bring dinner so that I wouldn't have to worry about cooking. While Allen wasn't a bad cook, they wanted to do something special for me as it was a custom send flowers or take food to someone not well or recovering to cheer them up. My friend, Elaine, brought a wonderful meal of chicken and dumplings, which really got my mouth watering once I got a whiff of it. While I wasn't sure what I could eat, I wanted to at least try to eat the gravy and maybe try a little bit of the dumplings also. I knew I wouldn't be able to eat the chicken, but the gravy and what little I had of the dumpling was delicious. It struck me how much you took food for granted until you found yourself restricted, and then you began to appreciate it so much more.

Allen and Sam ate while I entertained Elaine so I didn't have to watch them. I really enjoyed her company as I wasn't the type that liked to sit around at home. I was always career oriented and didn't enjoy being home so long from both maternity leave and the surgery. While many women preferred to be stay-at-home mothers, I was always the opposite and I was really beginning to miss work and the company of my friends. It was more than just the work; it was communicating with other adults and enjoying the accomplishments each day that brought satisfaction. I loved my family dearly, but I also appreciated myself as a woman and accepted that I wasn't cut out to be a homebody.

What was left over from dinner was enough for my lunch the next day. I had to train myself to visualize that the opening to my stomach was about the size am M&M candy, so I literally had to chew every almost to the point of liquid before swallowing. It was easier said than done, as like almost everyone, I had always chewed my food without thinking about it.

Sam was very curious about my new habits and asked Allen a number of questions. He wanted to know if I was sick and Allen told that I wasn't but that doctors and I had decided that the surgery would help me become a healthier person. Allen told him that I wouldn't be able to eat much anymore and that I also couldn't drink any sodas, but that I was fine and that everything would be back to normal in a few days.

That night before going to bed I was concerned about taking my antidepressant. It was the size of an M&M but I was really nervous about taking it, so I decided to break it in half before trying to swallow it. I did check with the pharmacist before the surgery and she told me that since the pills weren't time released there would be no problem breaking each tablet in half. Another challenge I faced was that I could no longer swallow large amounts of any liquid, including water, so I took half a tablet with a few small sips. I didn't quite manage to swallow the tablet and started worrying that it would start to dissolve and taste bitter.

I took a deep breath and tried swallowing again. Fortunately the tablet went down smoothly and I had no trouble with the second half now that I had a routine. Interestingly, I still had no real pain in my abdominal area, only some lower back discomfort.

***

The next morning, Chase woke me up around seven for a bottle. After I fed him I made some instant grits with butter for breakfast, but more runny than I was used to so I wouldn't have any problems swallowing it. I ate half and then stopped. For the next few days I ate grits, sugar free popsicles, jello and pudding. The nutrition list Dr. Reed provided suggested blending or straining foods, but it wasn't appealing. Broth wasn't much better, so I stuck to eating lots of jello and pudding.

I was also taking multivitamins, calcium and B-12 along with drinking 64 oz of water. Protein shakes helped cover my daily requirements, but since I couldn't drink the entire shake, I'd refrigerate the rest and have it later in the day. Because the shakes tasted somewhat like chocolate milk, they were easier to drink and didn't have such a chalky taste.

Since basketball season was starting up, I went to Sam's game on Saturday morning. I took my time walking, since I didn't want to trip or make any sudden movements that might strain the incisions. Allen carried Chase and I brought my sugar free breakfast shake. I wanted to drink the shake before the game was over so I at least finished one before I had to drink another. While I wasn't pushing myself hard, I did have a schedule I needed to maintain to ensure I got my daily requirement of protein and vitamins.

The following week I started experimenting with mashed potatoes, which had become my new favorite food. Broth or strained foods weren't working for me because I didn't think I was getting any nutritional value, nor did I honestly like them. Sugar free drinks mixed with water were fine, and I particularly enjoyed the lemonade and fruit punch flavors. While cream of wheat or oatmeal weren't on my favorites list, their soft consistencies became my breakfast of choice.

By the third week I started trying more meats, so I cooked a pork loin with potatoes and carrots. I started by eating some potatoes and then tried a small slice of pork. Not only was I practically getting a high from the aroma, but it was delicious even when I had to chew everything to a pulp. The only issue was that at one point I didn't chew the food as well as I should have, and boy, did I learn a very quick lesson there. This time it came up, and I just about made it to the bathroom. I doubt the food even reached my stomach, because I felt it about half way down my esophagus. I heard gurgling and then I felt a chill course through my body. It was a more an uncomfortable than a painful sensation, but after that experience I didn't want to eat meat anymore for a little while. One benefit is that my family was eating healthier along with me. Allen and Sam both loved mashed potatoes and pork loin.

    Next I tried scrambled eggs, low-fat cottage cheese, and sliced cheese, which worked well for me. Unfortunately, my attempt to eat a banana was another lesson in the importance of thorough chewing. I had assumed its mushy texture would be fine, but it was also thick, so once again, it came back up. At this point it was becoming difficult for me fulfill my required protein intake, even though I had a shake in the morning and tried eating eggs or cottage cheese on a regular basis. The shakes were a struggle to drink because most were chalky and not very tasty, and I was getting tired of the few I could tolerate.

    I recalled the support meetings I attended before my surgery when the speaker asked for a hand count of those who got their required daily protein. No one raised their hand. At the time I couldn't image why, as I thought it would be simple enough. Now I understood that it was quite a challenge when you had to focus so much only not only what you ate, but how much and how. The proof was in the two protein shots I'd purchased, one still untouched in the refrigerator. A few gulps and it was down, but somehow I couldn't seem to bring myself to drink it.

    What stood out the most about the meetings were the stories from those who had the surgery. One woman's story in particular really touched me. She had lost over 100 pounds and she felt great. But the most interesting part of her story was the amount of medications she was on before the surgery. Her health was rapidly declining due to high blood pressure, heart issues and other problems that actually threatened her life. She wasn't thin, perhaps a size 16, but the joy shining from her face had truly moved me, since not only did she feel and look great, but she could now play with her grandchildren. I knew by watching and listening to her that she was truly happy to be alive and that the surgery was a life-changing experience for her.

Another speaker that stood out at the meeting was a man that came in with such energy and excitement that I honestly though he had been drinking before he arrived. He loved being the center of attention and he couldn't stop talking about how proud he was that he lost over 100 pounds. This man was loving life and literally walked with a bounce in his step. I was just so amazed at how happy he was. He wasn't a small man either, perhaps a little larger than average, but if there was a success story to be told, it was definitely his.

While I was embarrassed to be at the meeting, I realized everyone there were ordinary, everyday people. No one judged me, and everyone was honest about their experiences before and after the surgery. Interestingly, it was the smaller things that many people missed, such as one woman missing a cold diet Coke poured into a glass of ice, or another woman wishing she had opted for the surgery at a younger age so her skin wouldn't have been as saggy afterward.

I continued to try different foods that I normally ate before surgery and some new ones too. It was time for my two week check up with Dr. Reed. I arrived just a few minutes before the appointment time. I had a completely different mindset from the first time I had an appointment with Dr. Reed. As I parked I was looking forward to seeing him and to find out how much weight I had lost. My incision where almost completely healed and I was doing great. I felt proud that not only had the surgery been successful, but all the months of preparation as well.

To say that I was proud of my accomplishments was an understatement. I had the Mt. Everest of my life on my own terms. No one bullied me or talked me into it, no one made me feel guilty about having the surgery. I followed through with all the research, seminars, appointments, and requirements. More importantly, I dealt with my fears of what others might think or say, and above all, my anxiety about the surgery.

I made the difficult decision for myself and my family, and I knew that my lifelong struggle with my weight was a battle I had finally won. It was my time to be a healthy person and enjoy life as God had planned for me. Now I could look in the mirror and see a different person, a better, healthier woman, wife and mother.

Chapter 7 - Triumphs and Challenges

      Since I had my surgery on November 10th, with Thanksgiving rapidly approaching I wasn't sure how I was going to handle it, so to make things easier, Allen and I decided to spend the holiday with his brother, Tommy, and his wife, Krystal, along with his paternal grandmother, various aunts, uncles, cousins and some friends. Since Tommy and Krystal had six children, they were excited to see us. They hadn't yet met Chase so we were excited to show off our latest addition. I made sure to bring some sugar free apple juice with me on the trip so I wouldn't have to worry about buying drinks at service areas or gas stations. This way I wouldn't be tempted by sodas or sugary drinks. Also, as much as I loved tea, the further north you traveled the more scarce it became, since sweet tea was more a southern tradition.

      As much as water sometimes got boring, because I drank so much of it my body now craved it. I also carried sugar free pudding for quick snacks in case I got hungry and there wasn't anything suitable to eat. A friend of my brother-in-law was concerned about me traveling for eight hours only two weeks after surgery, but I'd been feeling fine so I didn't think I'd have any issues. Steve also had the gastric bypass surgery about a year earlier and had mentioned some of the issues he'd experienced. About four hours into the trip I did feel some discomfort in my lower back but I took some pain medication and soon felt much better.

Meals ended up being the challenge for me, and again I learned some difficult lessons. While we got some fast food for lunch, my choices were extremely limited. Since I already had my apple juice I didn't feel bad about not ordering a soda like I normally would have done, but I did order off the child's menu. Well, that was a mistake as I'd only eaten two bites of the popcorn chicken before I started feeling sick. After eating ten fries I didn't want to eat anymore not only because I wasn't hungry but I also didn't want to get sick from eating fast food. It was a habit I was going to have to instill within me that I had to prepare better meals and snacks for traveling. I couldn't expect to find healthy choices at gas stations or service stops because that's not what these places catered to. Realistically, it was easier to get a burger and fries and be on your way. The problem was that I wasn't used to preparing meals or snacks beforehand because of time limitations, but if my diet was going to work I had to learn how to work around it. I also had to look at the benefits of healthier eating for my family. It wasn't about me anymore. We were all in this together.

A few more hours of driving brought us to dinner time. We didn't want to bother my in-laws because it was a weeknight and we didn't want them to come home from work and cook for us, so we stopped at a Chinese restaurant. I realized it was going to be a bad habit to break, but I thought I'd be fine with steamed rice and sautéed shrimp with only water to drink. I took my time and chewed really well ... or so I thought. After a few bites I got my now familiar chills and felt sick. I immediately looked for the restroom sign and without saying a word to my family, rushed past everyone praying that it wouldn't be a single stall and that it wouldn't be occupied, otherwise the consequences were going to be pretty grim.

Thankfully a woman had just finished and was coming out. I grabbed the door and ran in without even locking it. After a few minutes of regurgitating I felt better, but it took me a moment to calm down and regain my composure. I rinsed my mouth with water and blotted my face with a damp paper towel. I certainly felt much better than I had a few minutes ago. When I returned to the table Allen and Sam were worried about me asked if I was all right. I told them I was fine and left it at that. I felt neither hungry nor sick, but I knew that I couldn't eat anything else. As unpleasant as the episode was, it was simply a reminder that I had made a commitment that I had to stick to.

***

The honeymoon is over (3 months Post-Surgery). It's now been three months since my surgery. For the last three weeks I've maintained my 60 pound weight loss but haven't lost anymore. At least I haven't gotten sick for several weeks either, and I've been able to keep my food down and gradually increase the variety of foods as well. I finally started to learn that it was okay not to finish everything on my plate by gauging correct food portions. Now and again I still caught myself fixing a full plate of food and when I sat down to eat I realized that old habits really die hard. I had to train myself to accept that I could no longer eat all this food, but I could enjoy smaller portions that would still fill me up without feeling deprived. Bread plates have made it easier for me to control portions without the guilt of wasting food, and I still diligently took my vitamins and protein shakes, along with protein bars for snacks.

At least I managed to find a chocolate and nut protein bar that I really enjoyed. It tasted just like a candy bar so I started having one daily around three when I got a craving for something sweet. Not only was it good for me, but it saved me getting something from the vending machine at work and then getting funny looks from other employees who might wonder why I was eating candy so soon after weight loss surgery. No doubt I imagined reactions more than actually noticed them, but the thought of people talking about me worked wonders in keeping me away from the vending machines.

By now I had started drinking sweet tea again, which was my favorite drink. I ordered it half and half whenever we went to restaurants, and I found I enjoyed it just as much with less sugar. It had been a journey of trial and error getting used to my new eating habits, and my stomach never failed to let me know if I was eating more than it could handle by making some interesting sounds. It was almost like it was a separate entity living inside me because I had no control over the sounds. Sometimes it sounded like liquid going down a funnel and other times it sounds like I had gas.

That was one of the most embarrassing side effects of the surgery because my stomach constantly made sounds. While no one ever mentioned it, I knew people had to hear because I noticed it. I'm sure everyone assumed I had gas, but it was another incentive to watch how and what I ate because I didn't want people thinking that I had gas all the time. A number of people at the group meetings I had attended had mentioned that they suffered from bad gas after weight loss surgery, and I was grateful I at least hadn't fallen into that category. Whenever my stomach started getting noisy, I'd either do something like play with my jewelry or make some other noise to distract attention.

The only way to stop the noise was to eat less, which didn't mean depriving myself but eating less than I currently was. I certainly didn't want to stretch my stomach. After recently weighing myself I lost another 3.6 pounds so I had now lost a total of 63.6 pounds. While I was still making progress, I realized the honeymoon was over; I couldn't lose weight without trying anymore. I had to carefully watch what I ate and make the right choices.

Four months after my surgery people really started to notice the change. Whenever I went to the break room at work people complimented me on how great I looked. Even strangers who didn't know about my surgery asked what diet plan I used to lose weight. When I told them that I had weight loss surgery and have since changed my eating habits and have started exercising, they were really impressed. Others noticed but said nothing, and merely checked me out after noticing that I had lost weight. All in all it was a matter of maintenance, since Dr. Reed had cleared me and I was to call him if and when I needed him for any reason.

***

After five months I lost 73 pounds. I not only felt great but I noticed I had more energy and I became more active. I didn't mind parking further away and having to walk and I now walked to restaurants for lunch because my feet no longer hurt. I had started taking the stairs instead of the elevator and no longer got winded or uncomfortable. This was a real milestone for me and boosted my confidence to no end. Now I not only kept up with everyone else, I was in ever better shape than some of them.

Another great milestone for me was buying some new clothes because my old ones were starting to look baggy on me. Since my co-workers had started calling me 'droopy drawers' and tugged on my pants throughout the day. While it sure brought a smile to my face, I also didn't want to look like a clown at work, so I went to buy some new pants. I didn't know what size to try on so I got two different sizes. Imagine my surprise when I fit into the smaller of the two sizes and they fit beautifully. I was so excited I did a little celebration dance in the dressing room. I even looking for more clothes to try on and was having a wonderful time actually choosing what I liked instead of settling for whatever fit.

It was a day I never thought would come ... I could actually pick and choose clothes. I was no longer stuck with a limited choice and was no longer confined to plus size selections. I shopped for about two hours and tried on more clothes than I had for a long time before finally buying some that I actually loved. It was a great day for me and my self-esteem, and was a day I'd remember for the rest of my life.

When I got home I told Allen that I bought some new clothes and looked pretty damned good in them. He just smiled, congratulated me and asked me to model them. My confidence hit the ceiling that day and I found that I no longer worried about how my clothes looked or fit on me. Instead I could actually enjoy everything going on around me. Before, I was constantly self-conscious about how I looked, but because I was now comfortable in my new, attractive clothing, I no longer worried about how I looked, I was simply able to enjoy living in the moment.

***

The next turning point occurred when I went to see Dr. Powell for a routine visit. He was beyond delighted to see my progress since the surgery and wanted to know everything. In all the years I'd been a patient I had never seen him smile or change his tone of voice, but today he did. I could tell that he was truly happy for me and he wanted me to continue to improve myself. He told me that it was more than likely that I wouldn't need knee replacement surgery when I got older if I continued to lose weight and maintain it. I would also be more likely to avoid getting high blood pressure, diabetes, sleep apnea, and other obesity-related ailments, so he was delighted that I had opted for the surgery.

He did remind me to be careful and use preventative measures for birth control because a lot of women who lost weight found themselves more fertile and often became pregnant. I was aware of this and I did thank him for reminding me because I didn't want another child right now since Chase was only five months old.

I continued taking my vitamins, but I had come to notice that when I didn't get enough protein I lost more hair then normal while washing or blow drying. Once I returned to my required intake the hair loss stopped, which was a pretty strong reminder to continue consuming as much protein as possible. I ate cheese as snacks and tried to eat as much meat as possible. Bacon became my favorite food during this time, though I knew it wasn't the best choice. Still, I only ate a couple of pieces a week and considered it my treat, which was enough to satisfy me and not leave me feeling deprived.

Bread was something I still didn't find easy to eat, so I avoided it as much as possible. I was much more disciplined now about eating smaller portions and had gotten used to eating meals on a bread plate. It took some getting used to but now even Sam knew that the little plate was mine. I'd even started watching his portion sizes because I didn't want him to go through the same thing I had. If I started instilling good habits in him now, he wouldn't even notice and would grow up healthier.

***

After eight months I lost 92 pounds. My average weight loss was two pounds a week but sometimes I just maintained my weight. I'd started eating a little more than I had the last few months, but I still ate very little and didn't notice it much anymore. The only time I did notice how little I ate was when I went to a restaurant, and when the meal arrived the plate seemed so enormous. Compared to my bread plate sized meal, restaurants servings looked like platters. Obviously I knew I couldn't possibly eat so much so I sampled small potions and tried to balance them so I would be satisfied nutritionally and emotionally. It was never junk food, and each time I chose potatoes over bread.

    I still wasn't eating that much bread. I was never a big bread eater anyway, and on the occasion I did have some, it filled me up fast and I didn't feel like I had a healthy meal. It was just filler and I didn't feel satisfied. Again, it was the lesson of making better choices. One of the things that I thought I'd have difficulty with after the surgery was not controlling my hunger and binge eating, but I found that I'd gotten quite accustomed to eating only small amounts. I still got full like I did before the surgery, but with less food.

    On the rare occasion that I did overeat, my stomach reminded me in no uncertain terms that I still hadn't fully learned my lesson. Interestingly, my taste for certain foods changed as well. I no longer cared for processed meat anymore, though at one time my favorite food was hot dogs or Polish sausages. I'd loved them since I was a child, but after trying a little I became so sick I never ate them again.

    My cooking habits also changed to heartier, more nutritious meals that satisfied my hunger. My favorites were potatoes, beans, cheeses, soups, vegetables, and fruits. I'd lost my taste for heavy or overly sweet food. I did see a reoccurrence of hair loss because I slacked off on my vitamins, and finding more hair in the shower or on my clothes was one way to get me back on track.

    Another habit I had to adopt was making sure I ate at more regular intervals as I'd started to notice myself getting lightheaded from waiting too long between meals. A friend who also had the surgery mentioned this, so I got into the habit of snacking more often to avoid letting my blood sugar drop.

    My colleagues, as well as people I saw locally, continued to ask about my weight loss. Their interest not only boosted my confidence but kept me motivated to keep going until I reached my goal, which was nice to no longer be a plus size. I wasn't targeting a particular amount of weight to lose, I simply wanted to wear normal size clothes and never have to visit the plus size or women's section of a store again. Funny thing, I always thought that 'W' in plus size clothes meant 'wide,' not 'women'. I'd overheard some friends of mind talking about the difference between these sizes, and somehow I assumed that's what 'W' meant. Needless to say I was relieved to learn otherwise.

    The best thing about losing 92 pounds was that I could actually cross my legs. It was awkward before, but now I could be ladylike about it. For most people it wasn't a big deal, but it was another milestone for me because I'd never been able to comfortably cross my legs. Now I could, and I could do it without even thinking about it. When I realized I could do this it just made my heart smile. This simple action was one of the most gratifying things the surgery provide me, and I was slowly returning to the woman inside people never saw before because of my weight.

    I was also proud of how I stopped drinking any soda or carbonated beverage. It didn't matter that there was nothing else to drink. If that was the case I simply drank water. Yes, there were times I was tempted to drink a cold, refreshing Coke, but I resisted. I wasn't going to risk everything I had accomplished but returning to old habits. While I still drank sweet tea, it wasn't carbonated and I added the least amount of sugar possible. I was proud of myself for going nine months without even a sip of a carbonated beverage. Thank goodness I wasn't a beer drinker, as that would have been forbidden as well.

***

    Recently I started considering a tummy tuck, but I didn't yet feel I was ready for it. I still wanted to lose more weight, plus it had only been nine months since the surgery. I still had plenty of time to shed more pounds and then maintain my weight before dealing with a tummy tuck. My arms were really the worst part of my body and I had some bat wings going on right now, and it wasn't likely that any amount of exercise would bring those puppies back to life. I still avoided sleeveless tops and the only way anyone was going to glimpse my upper arms was if I wore a bathing suit at the river or pool. They weren't a pretty sight so until I got reduction surgery, they'd remain out of sight for now.

Monday was my usual weigh-in day. I learned that weighing myself several times a week was too discouraging. People constantly asked why I didn't check more often, but it's impossible to lose weight every day. It wasn't only unhealthy for my body, but I felt I that losing a pound or two a week was a manageable pace. I wasn't about to become so obsessed with my weight that it consumed my every thought, I just wanted to be healthy and enjoy life. I knew what pace worked for me, and it wasn't necessary for me to abide by what other people thought I should be doing.

I did notice another issue related to my weight loss that never crossed my mind. When I went out to lunch with colleagues or there was food at a meeting, they often got uncomfortable with how little I ate. They undoubtedly felt self-conscious because they were eating larger portions than me. Some people asked if that was all I was eating or whether I was okay with the food because I ate very little. It became necessary to remind them that I couldn't eat much anymore because I got full very quickly. One trick I learned was to play with my food to make it look like I was eating more than I actually was. I never wanted to make anyone else feel bad about themselves because I didn't eat as much as they did, and frankly, I didn't really watch what and how much others ate. I just enjoyed their company and concentrated on my meal to ensure I chewed properly and didn't get sick. I didn't judge the eating habits of others because I had to deal with my own.

Apart from teaching myself new eating habits, I hadn't really experienced any real physical or emotional fallout from the surgery. I supposed I was fortunate because I had always been a positive, upbeat person. While I wasn't sure why it was necessary for me to undergo a psychiatric evaluation as part of the approval process, I assumed that some people might have a problem with the extreme changes weight loss surgery incurred on all levels of your life, which would be further complicated by problems existing before the surgery. For me, the surgery was a positive experience.

It was especially encouraging to have people compliment me on how good I looked or how well I'd progressed over the last few months. I absolutely loved that I was more active without getting out of breath or easily tired. Now I didn't have to worry about going places and having difficult with the seating or I would have to tackle stairs. I could enjoy my new clothes without worrying about my fat rolls showing. While I still had them, they were much smaller and they became benchmarks of my goal to become healthier and happier. Being able to actually enjoy life without worrying about my appearance and what people thought of me was not only a gift, it opened the door for me to experience life as I should, and to me, that was my definition of success.

Success also meant continually educating myself about food and my attitudes toward it. I was still testing the waters with certain foods, and had found that I couldn't tolerate heavier foods such as biscuits, steak, chicken, bananas, dressing, and turkey. Softer textures worked better for me and it was a while before I could really eat more meat, which helped greatly with my weight loss.

Now that I had lost 105 pounds I was really seeing and feeling the difference. Often at work I overheard others that didn't know about surgery talking about how great I looked and wondering how I lost so much weight. Of course I just smiled and pretended I didn't hear anything. One day while I was in the break room I overheard some women talking about how pretty I was, and that I had a beautiful face that just glowed now. I actually felt emotional, and even though they hadn't meant me to hear their conversation, it was a wonderful affirmation of my progress.

More and more people were curious and interested in how the surgery worked and what I had done, so I became an educator of sorts and gave them condensed versions that both answered their questions without completely grossing them out. Ironically, several colleagues approached me and asked specific questions because they were very interested in having the same surgery.

***

For the past couple of months I noticed I hadn't lost any weight, so I realized I probably had to change my diet to jump start my metabolism since my body had adjusted to the new food I was eating. I had fallen into a routine of eating the same things so it was time to become more creative and explore other healthy and tasty food choices. Once I made some changes to my diet I started losing weight again.

I still didn't eat much meat or bread. Sometimes I'd take a bite from a juicy cheeseburger, but my stomach never failed to remind me that it wasn't happy with my choice. Of course I fantasized about eating a burger or a slice of pizza, but the actual experience was never as good as my imagination. The fat never failed to upset my stomach and it was impossible to take a large bite of anything. No matter what I ate had to be chewed to a pulp, and if it took too long the effort just wasn't worth it as there was no satisfaction in it. At the back of my mind I also knew there was a good chance that I still might not chew properly or that the fat would make me sick. I'd rather have a healthy meal that satisfied me and I felt good afterward than risking another race to the bathroom. So my experiences really changed my perspective on what to eat.

Also, I had a habit of slacking off on my vitamins, so I decided to keep them by my contact lens solution so I remembered to take them. I wanted to look good as well as feel good, and healthy habits were the only ones I wanted from this point.

I continued to make changes in my meal planning and some were good and some not so good. There were a few meals that I prepared that just got tossed in the trash and others we absolutely loved it. I've definitely become a healthier cook and I'm more knowledgeable about the different types of food groups and have experimented with recipes I would have never tried before. By summertime I had lost 125 pounds and I was excited about getting a bathing suit. No, I didn't look like a supermodel, but I was comfortable in my own skin and even more so with my attitude. It was going to be a great summer, and I was looking forward to it!

Chapter 8 - Aftermath

    I'd been feeling some discomfort in my stomach area for a few weeks that occurred mainly when I stood up. It wasn't really painful when I sat down but whenever I got up I felt a twinge on my right side. At first I thought it might be my body readjusting to the new pouch, but to be on the safe side I decided to see Dr. Jones to get it checked out. I suspected that I might have another cyst on my fallopian tube, which I had when I was a teenager, so if that was the diagnosis, I knew it would entail another outpatient surgery and I'd be done with it.

    Needless to say I was more than concerned when Dr. Jones told me that he detected a mass in that area and ordered an ultrasound for the next day. My mind starting racing with all kinds of thoughts, and I wondered if I had some kind of tumor but he didn't want to say anything until he was sure. I prayed that it was only a cyst that could be quickly removed and then I would be fine. I did my best not to worry, but whose imagination wouldn't have worked overtime after that? I'd already been through my share of anxiety with the weight loss surgery and now I faced yet another challenge.

Allen asked if I wanted him to go with me to the appointment, but I told him it wasn't worth missing a day. He worked for the water department and he was one of only two staff in that department. His colleague was an older man about to retire, so Allen was conscientious about not missing work unless it was a scheduled vacation or one of the kids was sick and I couldn't take time off. When I returned to work after my lunchtime appointment with Dr. Jones, my close coworkers wanted to know how everything went. It was difficult to speak without crying. By now I was becoming more anxious and asked them to pray for me that it wouldn't be anything serious and that I would be fine.

When I returned to Dr. Jones' office the next day, Mary, the ultrasound technician, called me into a quiet room with soft music playing. That was her normal working environment and it was quite a relaxing atmosphere. By this point I was so nervous I was on the verge of tears. Mary, on the other hand, was the picture of calmness, an attractive brunette about 5'8 with a shoulder-length bob. It was evident that she enjoyed her job, and her demeanor helped calm me as she confirmed why I was there. I told her that the discomfort occurred only intermittently on my right side. I also updated her on my history so that she would know what to look for.

It was difficult to keep quiet during the ultrasound, but after several minutes I couldn't help myself and finally asked Mary if she saw anything. When she said that she did, my heart literally leapt into my mouth until she told me that it wasn't anything bad at all. She asked me if I wanted to take a look, so I thought even if I didn't know what I was looking at, I would at least feel better.

Imagine my shock when Mary turned the monitor toward me and pointed to a specific spot on the screen displaying a head and spine. All I could do was stare blankly at the image, then I glanced at the top left corner to make sure I saw my name and not someone else's. It was my name, so there was no mistake. Mary noticed how stunned I looked and asked if I was all right. I mumbled that I was, but then she smiled and said, "You didn't know."

When I shook my head, she told me that I was twelve weeks pregnant and everything looked fine. She printed out copies to share with my family, and suggested I take my time getting ready as she needed to fill out some paperwork. After I returned to the waiting room, Dr. Jones called me in to review the results. He confirmed that I was twelve weeks pregnant and gave me some vitamins to start taking. I was still in a state of shock as I truly had no clue I was pregnant! I serious thought I had a cyst or cancer. It never crossed my mind that I could have been pregnant. Chase was only fifteen-months old and I never thought about having a third child. I hadn't planned on this and I certainly wasn't expecting to have any more children in the near future; perhaps in a couple of years but not when I already had a baby. I did have the presence of mind to tell Dr. Jones that I had already been taking two multivitamins for a while now, and he said that was fine. He did express concern that I didn't look very happy about the news, which was an understatement.

All I could think about was that I would have two children in daycare, two in diapers, and two in car seats. Allen paid the daycare fees and it took 20% of his weekly pay, plus we provided diapers, snacks, etc. It was an amount were could afford, and we still had enough to cover and we were comfortable paying this amount. We were still comfortable buying groceries, gas and other necessities, including whatever Sam needed for school and sports. With another child in daycare, I knew Allen would lose anywhere from an extra 20-40% of his weekly check. Not only was our finances a concern, but even more was how I was going to cope with two small children.

How was I going to feel chasing Chase around while pregnant? Would I be able to handle it? Would my restricted diet have affected the baby's development? All I could think about was how my weight loss surgery might affect my pregnancy. It was like I was having a debate with ten people in my mind.

Dr. Jones suggested I sat in his office until I felt better, but my head was swimming from the shock of learning I was pregnant. He was concerned because I looked so pale and worried. I suppose he didn't want me hurting myself because I was inattentive or distracted. On the plus side, at least the diagnosis wasn't anything that I feared, but now I faced a different kind of worry.

I started thinking about our three-bedroom home, mid-size car and yet another maternity leave I would have to take from work. When I had calmed down enough, I told Dr. Jones that I felt better and that I was going back to work. He asked again if I felt up to driving, and I told I did, but when I got to the car I just sat there for a while thinking over and over again that I was pregnant. The irony was very apparent, especially after the difficulty I had getting pregnant with Chase.

We used the precautions that we had for years, which worked great for us. We had a strong marriage and our sex life improved after my surgery because I felt so much better about myself, but the reality was that neither of us expected that I would become pregnant so easily. Above all, I was also concerned about the financial strain on our relationship.

Finally, I felt settled enough to call Allen. I knew he'd be waiting for my call and was just as anxious as I'd been. So rather than call while I was on the road I called him from the parking lot.

I'll never forget the sound of his voice when I told him. First there was silence, and then he thought I was joking, but I confirmed that we really were going to have another baby. Once Allen realized that I was serious, he was as shocked as I was, but at the same time we were also excited. It certainly explained why I hadn't lost any weight in the last few weeks. I thought it was because I was in a rut and eating the same foods every day, but being pregnant was actually the last thing that would have crossed my mind.

I was far from ready to announce that I was pregnant again and was more than a little nervous about returning to work because I knew my co-workers would want to know what the doctor said. It was something I had yet to fully accept, and I wasn't equipped to deal with the reactions and inevitable comments from others.

After calling Allen I call Amelia. Even though she no longer worked with me we remained friends and talked often. As soon as she answered the phone I started crying. Amelia had three children and her third child had also been unplanned, which she called an unexpected blessing. I was finally able to express my concerns and fears. Not only did she understand completely, but she comforted me and made me feel so much at ease. At one point she was actually giggling because she was happy and knew exactly what I was going through.

I told her that I really didn't want to go back to work that afternoon and she suggested that I call my supervisor and tell them that I wasn't feeling well after the appointment and needed to go home. It wasn't technically a lie, so I followed her suggestion. Since it was Thursday, I knew I had one more day of work then I would have the weekend to come to terms with everything. Amelia assured me everything would work out fine and told me to call her back if I needed her regardless of the time. She was a wonderful friend and I not only learned a lot from her, but she helped me grow in my career and as a person. I knew she would always be there for me. I'm very thankful to have someone like her in my life.

***

When I returned to work on Friday I told everyone that I had to wait the doctor got the test results, which bought me time to think about my situation. I knew that my surgery wouldn't affect my ability to have children, and that being pregnant wouldn't affect my long-term weight loss goals, but the unexpected news put a different perspective on so many things that I was simply unprepared for. My co-workers were satisfied with my explanation, so at least I didn't have to field questions and comments about being pregnant again.

On Saturday, Chase and I were home by ourselves since Allen had taken Sam fishing at one of the ponds. I was trying to occupy my mind by cleaning and rearranging furniture but I couldn't deal with the noise in my head. I had to talk to someone else the news, so I took at break and emailed my friend Julie to see if she had time to talk. She had called because she knew I had a doctor's appointment on Thursday.

The moment she answered the phone I immediately started crying. I was overwhelmed and scared by the prospect of having another baby so soon after Chase, but she responded the same as Amelia and assured me that I was a great mother, and because I had done all the research about having a baby after the surgery, everything would be fine for me and the baby.

After our conversation I felt a lot better. I was grateful to have such a wonderful support system ... my husband, family and friends. I couldn't ask for anything more than that. When I went back to work on Monday, I decided to tell my co-workers about the news and apologized for not telling them about it on Friday. Everyone understood and congratulated me on the wonderful news. I became emotional and started crying because I was so overwhelmed. There was nothing like having a child in your life, and I realized that they were miracles and that I was blessed with yet another one. I prayed and gave all my concerns to Jesus, and asked him to guide me through the next chapter of my life.

***

After a few more weeks of pregnancy, it was time to discover the sex of the baby. I had another appointment with Mary to have an ultrasound to ensure the baby was growing properly. During the procedure Mary confirmed that I was having a girl. I was so excited I could barely contain myself; two boys, and now a girl. Mary and I were smiling from ear to ear. She confirmed that everything looked great and I was on track to having a healthy baby girl.

Once again I only gained nine pounds during my pregnancy, which was the same weight that I gained the previous times. As before, I experienced morning sickness, and while my eating habits remained the same during my pregnancy, the morning sickness helped keep my weight down. It wasn't intentional, but that's how it worked out so at least weight gain wasn't a major concern.

My daughter Elizabeth was born the day before my birthday. She was a healthy baby. I had no complications with the pregnancy beyond some difficulty with my blood sugar test. Because I had to drink a very sweet liquid within a certain amount of time, I found I couldn't hold down enough liquid in my pouch so it quickly came back up. I had to reschedule the test and try it a different way. Fortunately, Lisa, Dr. Jones' nurse, suggested that I bring jelly beans to try next time and I passed with flying colors.

***

As time went on I continued to feel great. While I noticed that I was still losing some hair, I also started seeing regrowth since I started sticking with my vitamin and higher protein intake. However, it seemed that while I was losing weight, Allen was gaining it because he started eating all the food I didn't so it wouldn't go to waste. We quickly realized what was going on so I became more stringent about controlling my portions so there wouldn't be leftovers to tempt Allen. The last thing I wanted was to see him develop a weight problem.

Maintaining my weight wasn't the chore I thought it would be and I was enjoying everything about it. Since I started feeling better and able to get around much easier I started walking more for exercise. After a few weeks home with Elizabeth, summer was in full swing and it was getting hot and muggy as was typical for that region, so I decided it was time to go shopping for a new bathing suit since I'd lost so much weight. It was certainly strange for me to enjoy shopping for clothes because for so long it was a horrible experience and always reminded me how overweight I was. Now that I could shop for cute outfits instead of what could fit into, it had become a pleasure.

I was able to buy such cute bathing suits for Elizabeth, and I was more than excited that I could finally wear something stylish and attractive. My sister-in-law Marie had a pool so Elizabeth and I took full advantage of hanging out by the pool while I was on maternity leave. Of course we stayed in the shade since she was still only a few weeks old but I enjoyed my alone time with her every chance I could. I took photos of us together out by the pool and shared them with friends and co-workers. This was something new for me as I never would have taken pictures of myself in a bathing suit, let alone send them to anyone. This new level of confidence was just another milestone for me and I could now enjoy life without worrying so much about how I looked. The Fourth of July week was around the corner and we were getting ready to head to Missouri for our family vacation, which had a beautiful river and recreational area.

***

After having Elizabeth, I lost an additional 15 pounds. Within eight weeks after giving birth I was lost another 15 pounds, bringing my total weight loss to date down to 135 pounds. Better yet, I was down another two sizes. My best friend was getting married, which gave me the perfect reason to buy a new outfit for the wedding. While shopping, I was more than delighted to find that the size I wore before I was pregnant was too big, so I tried on a smaller size. Once again I was grinning like a madwoman. I'm sure people where staring at me, but who cared? No more plus sizes for me, I was wearing average sizes and I was jazzed. I did my little dance in the dressing room again, and I was so excited I wanted to scream. I'd dreamed about this for so long, and now it was finally happening. I was wearing extra large now and I couldn't believe it!

My weight loss was becoming more and more obvious in ways other than wearing smaller sizes. When I went out to eat with friends they noticed how little I ate. Some people seemed uncomfortable and would ask if I was all right, and I patiently explained the situation, but by now most people I regularly ate with knew or had gotten used to my habits.

A normal selection for me was meat, a couple of vegetables, and cornbread, which I usually never finished. I often took the leftovers home because I knew I wasn't going to clean my plate and I never wanted to waste food. But my friends still not only asked if that was all I was having, but why I wasn't finishing my meal. It was an interesting study in perceptions because people really paid attention to how little I ate, as opposed to how much I ate before. Perhaps it was because I made others feel they were eating too much, but I never really paid attention to the eating habits of others. My concern was eating the correct portions for me and taking the leftovers home.

I never would have thought my eating habits would affect others so much, but even after almost two years they still asked the same questions. In the beginning it was somewhat of a trial and error process to judge correct portions for me, but over time it became second nature. Even on the road, I ordered from the child's menu and only ate some of it. The only problem was that the meals usual came with a small drink, which I never drank. Beyond that, the child's portion was the perfect amount of food even if I shared some of my fries with my toddler. I still didn't each much bread, but I did order cornbread sometimes and pick at it because I liked it. On the rare occasions when I ordered a burger I never ate all the bun, at most, maybe half and the inside, which I considered the good stuff. Breakfast was the same, I ate mostly the filling in the biscuit instead of the biscuit itself. I tended to find crunchier foods easier to manage than softer and thicker foods, and trial and error had finally taught me what to eat as I hadn't been sick from improperly chewing for quite some time.

***

While we were enjoying our family vacation camping, barbecuing, and swimming, I began experiencing sharp pains in my right side that seemed to focus under my ribs and around my back. At first the discomfort was only occasional, but after it increased, I realized I was facing yet another situation with my health. Allen and I were taking the kids to the lake so Sam could swim and Chase and Elizabeth could just hang out under the shade and roll around on the blanket. There was a lovely grassy park edging the lake that offered the perfect setting for relaxing by the water.

We were really looking forward to our day out, but as we drove there, Allen made a joke, and when I laughed I felt a very sharp pain resonate from my side. I told him that it wasn't a severe pain, but it was definitely uncomfortable. I knew that I hadn't hurt myself because I hadn't picked up anything heavy or done anything strenuous enough to pull a muscle. It simply flared up and eased off.

The discomfort was enough to put me off eating and that alarmed Allen. I noticed him watching me to make sure I ate something later that day, but I just didn't have the appetite for it. Finally I told him that I wanted to make an appointment with Dr. Powell for a checkup. When I saw him, he suggested an ultrasound because he suspected I might have gallstones. Sure enough, the test revealed that I did indeed have them. When Dr. Powell scheduled an appointment with the surgeon, I requested Dr. Reed since I was his patient and he regularly performed gallstone surgery.

Interestingly, when I asked Dr. Powell about gallstones, he determined that rapid weight loss could often cause them. This was something I wasn't aware of before I had my surgery, and while I knew a few people who had their gallbladders removed, I never made the connection. Now I had done a considerable amount of research for my surgery, but I couldn't remember finding anything about gallstones as a result of weight loss surgery.

Then I thought about it some more and I did recall one support meeting I attended where the speaker asked how many attendees required gallbladder surgery after having weight loss surgery. Though half the audience raised their hands, I never gave it any further thought until Dr. Powell mentioned it. After my appointment I went home and researched weight loss surgery and gall bladder problems. Sure enough, that perfectly described my condition.

I learned that my gallbladder was a small organ near my liver. It released bile, a digestive fluid, into the bile duct, which fed into the small intestine. Rapid weight loss, align with other risk factors, often caused gallstones, which were small pieces of hardened material that blocked the flow of bile and caused pain and other symptoms. Rapid weight loss was one factor in their development because as the body burned fat more quickly, some of the cholesterol in the liver seeped into the bile, which could cause cholesterol gallstones. Repeated weight gain and loss were primary risk factors, but also a diet high in fat and cholesterol, family history and a diagnosis of diabetes. People over the age of sixty were more likely to develop gallstones, along with women and those taking cholesterol-lowering medications. So there it was ... yet another interesting byproduct of rapid weight loss.

I had an appointment scheduled with Dr. Reed a week later. The pain wasn't constant, but it was erratic and often very uncomfortable. After talking to Dr. Reed he immediately recognized the problem and assured me that this issue was common so there was no need to be alarmed. He was as calm as always, eased my concerns and told me that he could used the same access points that he had for the bypass surgery. He also prescribed some pain medication until I had the procedure, which was a quick outpatient surgery scheduled for the next morning. I'd be on my way home after a few hours. Allen was worried that I was going to have yet another surgery but I assured him that I wasn't planning on anything else anytime soon and this couldn't be helped.

The next morning Allen and I arrived at the hospital at 9:30am. It was the same place I had my bypass surgery so I knew the routine. After filling out the paperwork and paying a $250 co-payment, the receptionist put on my wrist band and told me to wait until someone called my name. A few minutes later a nurse led us back to a room where I changed into a gown. Allen sat beside the bed while the nurse started the IV and made sure I was ready to go.

It was nothing like the gastric bypass surgery. This time I was lying in the bed watching TV and waiting to be taken into surgery without the anxiety and stress that I experienced before. I had completely confidence in Dr. Reed and the hospital staff. The removal of the my gall bladder took less than an hour to have the actually procedure. It did add an inch-long scar right above my belly button to my other trophies, but it wasn't that big of a deal and I was fine after a couple of days of rest. It occurred to me that I'd never asked how many stones I had or how large they were, but I suppose I didn't want to get too grossed out.

About a week after the surgery, I quickly noticed that I couldn't eat eggs or any fatty foods. Dr. Reed didn't mention anything about watching my diet and I don't remember the release nurse mentioning it either. If she did, I must have missed it. This new restriction to my diet became painfully apparent when Allen and I went to a barbecue and I ate a hamburger patty with ketchup. I had barely swallowed it when I started experiencing sharp stomach pain. At first I wasn't sure what had happened because I had thoroughly chewed the burger, but the fat was too much for my body to handle since breaking down fat had been the purpose of the gallbladder. Without it, anything fatty would upset my stomach.

Though the pain only lasted about twenty minutes, I couldn't finish my dinner. Allen and my brother-in-law, Tommy, immediately noticed that something was wrong and asked if I was all right. I told them I didn't know because my stomach was really hurting. I told them that I thought I chewed everything well but something was going on and I didn't know what it was. I decided not to try anything else until the next morning, when I attempted to eat some breakfast sausage. Unfortunately, even though I tried absorbing as much fat as possible after cooking it, it also upset my stomach.

I also found myself on quite a regular bathroom run, which was another byproduct of gallbladder removal. Now I faced even more restrictions with my diet as I'd lost my taste for many foods because they upset my stomach. At times it was frustrating because I needed to maintain my protein intake, and the problem was that I could no longer tolerate many of those foods, meat, in particular. Sometimes I pushed the limits even though I knew it would upset my stomach, and occasionally I got away with it.

My stomach continued to make interesting growling sounds if I ate too much, and they were far from quiet as well. It was embarrassing for me and if I felt others heard it while we were talking I simply apologized and carried on. This was also an effective deterrent to keep me from over-eating because I certainly didn't want my stomach making strange noises at inopportune moments. My stomach also growled a lot if I ate too soon before going to bed. It was always louder at night and Allen joked that it sounded like I was growling at him.

For now I couldn't seem to control or stop it, but I continued to make adjustments in my diet in the hopes that it would eventually stop. It wasn't uncomfortable, it was simply a growling that lasted anywhere from five to fifteen minutes before it stopped. I did conduct some additional research to see if this was also a byproduct of the surgery and discovered that the sounds were my digestive system processing the food. Several people mentioned it and also commented that the noise got worse at night. No one complained of any discomfort, only that it could be embarrassing at times and that there was way to control it.

It was an annoying but minor issue and wouldn't have affected my decision to undergo the surgery. The benefits I had reaped by losing a significant amount of weight far outweighed the smaller issues and inconveniences, and with patience and perseverance, I knew I'd find a way to deal with this as well.

***

Since going back to work after Elizabeth's birth, I gained seven pounds because I wasn't preparing snacks for myself like I did while I was at home. After I noticed myself heading to the vending machine again I started bringing sugar free pudding, bananas and cheese for snacks. That alone brought me down three pounds in just one week. Most importantly I still avoided carbonated drinks. I admit there were times I was tempted, but I always resisted. Instead, I stuck with sweet tea, sugar-free fruit punch and water. While the sound of a soda can popping open still evoked fond memories, it was also a reminder why I had gained so much weight, and I knew I wasn't going back down that road again.

Eight months after returning to work I gradually gained twenty-two pounds. While I still wasn't eating much, I was eating less healthy food as I had started visiting the vending machines again. When I felt my clothes getting tighter it was a wakeup call, as there was no way I was going back to plus sizes. I started bringing healthy snack items to work again, such as hard candy, pretzels, and gum. Sometimes when I was busy at work I just wanted something to munch on, so I ate cottage cheese, yogurt and other filling foods to help keep me going until lunch or dinner. At 10:00 and 3:00 I had a snack, which helped stabilize my blood sugar so I wouldn't feel faint and be tempted to eat unhealthy snacks.

I realized that I sometimes suffered from the effects of 'Dumping syndrome,' which was a common side effect of gastric bypass surgery that occurred when the contents of the stomach move too quickly through the small intestine and caused nausea, weakness, fainting, sweating and diarrhea. Foods high in sugar or fat typically caused these symptoms, so it was yet another reason for me to try and avoid these items.

People continued to notice how much weight I had lost and complimented me on how great I looked.

On Valentine's Day, our department had planned to have a food day at work, which we called a potluck because everyone brought something for the staff to eat throughout the day. A friend of mine, Alisa, had just started baking cakes and candies on the side to help bring some extra income in for her family, so I asked her to make a candy tray for me to bring. That way I was helping her out and she was helping me out by making something homemade to take to work. It was awesome and everyone loved it. I grabbed a few pieces myself and set them on a plate on my desk so I had enough to satisfy me without going back to be tempted by all the delicious food.

Throughout the day, producers brought job requests and noted the completion times. One particular producer came by to hand me a job request. James was a short, small framed man who didn't mind sharing his opinion about whether invited or not. As he was describing what needed to be done for the presentation, he admonished me for eating the treats because I'd been doing so well on my diet. His attitude irritated me because I didn't need someone preaching to me, so I let him know that I didn't appreciate being lectured on what to eat. Unfortunately, he didn't seem to take the hint and further suggested that he should come to my desk and police what I ate. I laughed and told him that it wasn't a good idea, hoping he'd get the message this time.

When I sent the document to print, I told him to wait by the center printer, but I followed him to ensure everything was printing correctly. Lo and behold, I caught him scarfing down a handful of chips. The look on his face was priceless. I laughed at the irony, and he had no choice but to laugh at himself.

So it was yet another lesson I learned about human nature during my journey with weight loss. Most people are supportive, while some won't say anything at all or will say the wrong things. I suppose it had to do with their comfort levels, or perhaps facing their own issues.

Obesity has become a national problem, and the health ramifications reach far and wide. It's no longer an individual issue, but an issue that affects those around you. No matter what your size or budget, if you want to do something about losing weight, do your homework and learn about your options and which one is right for you. You don't have to tell anyone until you're ready to make a decision, and above all, make your own decision based on what's right for you, your body, and your health.

There are many factors to consider beyond the preparation and the actual surgery. Above all, you must understand and accept that you're in this for life. If you decide halfway that this isn't the solution for you, that's fine. Don't let others dictate to you. There are no time limits on making serious decisions like this, but for me it was one of the best decisions I've ever made. I'm proud that I did my homework and took time to consider my decision without feeling rushed or pressured.

It was, and still is, an emotional process, and my ultimate goal was to be a better, healthier woman, wife, and mother. I'm now at a healthy weight and I'm teaching my family better eating habits so that they will hopefully never have to endure what I did. I can proudly say that I accomplished my goal by losing weight and becoming a better person for it.

Allen had always told me that I was beautiful, but now I also saw a beautiful woman in the mirror.

4/369.00
203 7855714
Laura

Made in the USA
Middletown, DE
02 March 2019